A QUICK TING ON...

THE BLACK GIRL AFRO

ZAINAB KWAW-SWANZY

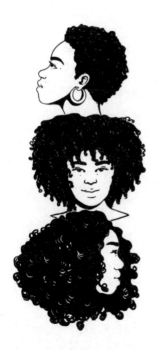

AQ
TO

JACARANDA

This edition first published in Great Britain 2022
Jacaranda Books Art Music Ltd
27 Old Gloucester Street,
London WC1N 3AX
www.jacarandabooksartmusic.co.uk

A CIP catalogue record for this book is available from the British
Library

Interviews edited for clarity and concision.

ISBN: 9781913090593
eISBN: 9781913090609

Cover Illustration: Camilla Ru
Cover Design: Baker, bplanb.co.uk
Typeset by: Kamillah Brandes

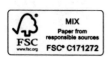

ALHAMDULILLAH.

TO MY ANGELIC BABY NIECE, YARA, AND THE FUTURE GENERATIONS OF KWAW-SWANZYS YET TO COME. I HOPE THAT ONE DAY YOU CAN READ THIS BOOK AND FEEL EMPOWERED AND EDUCATED!

THIS IS FOR EVERY YOUNG BLACK GIRL, PAST, PRESENT AND FUTURE, WHO STRUGGLED WHILST NAVIGATING THEIR HAIR JOURNEYS. YOU AND YOUR HAIR ARE BEAUTIFUL, NO MATTER WHAT.

CONTENTS

PREFACE

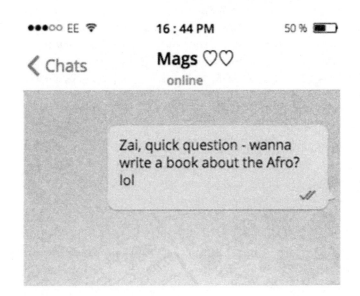

●●●○○ EE 📶   **16 : 44 PM**   50 % 🔋

‹ Chats   **Mags** ♡♡
                        online

Zai, quick question - wanna
write a book about the Afro?
lol

This was how my friend Mags asked me to be part of
her *A Quick Ting On* book series. My phone repeatedly
buzzed as each Whatsapp message came through with voice
notes. In them, Mags detailed the concept of the series and
how me and my afro could fit in. To date, it is probably one of
the most surprising Whatsapp messages I have ever received.

I'll be honest, my first thought was a strong no. Me? Write
a book? I mean yes, I've written articles and short pieces in the
past, but a whole book? That was a totally different ball game.

If I am honest, writing a book about Afro hair was always a dream, but it was an opportunity that I never thought I would have access to. Then, in true serendipitous form, Mags messages me out of the blue. Before I could answer cohesively, Mags sent me some voice notes and after playing each one, I began to feel more encouraged, more confident and so incredibly grateful to be asked to write about a topic that I am so passionate about. My journey with my hair, like many Black women, has been long, complex, meaningful and beautiful and because of this, this is the book I was always meant to write.

Before we begin, I want to discuss what I mean when I say Afro hair, the afro, or Afro-textured hair. The afro is commonly recognised as a hairstyle where Black hair is left out in its natural state and often appears kinky or tight curled, commonly growing in an elevated manner all around the scalp. Over the course of this book, I will also make reference to 'natural hair', which is hair not altered by chemicals. Another term that will appear often will be 'Black hair', which refers to the hair of Black people, rather than hair that is black in colour.

The term 'Afro', however, is not exclusive to hair only. In fact, the prefix 'Afro-' has a far wide ranging definition, and one that provides more depth to the meaning of 'Afro hair'. The prefix 'Afro-' means 'of African descent ' or 'African'. We see this in the multiple words that include the prefix, from Afrofuturism, which relates to futuristic or scientific themes which incorporate Black and African history and culture, to Afrobeats, which is a genre of music originating from West Africa. Oddly, mainstream definitions of Afro hair make no mention of Blackness or Africaness, and almost suggest that anyone can have Afro hair if they just style and shape it in the right way, but this is not true. Afro hair is scientifically different to the straight or wavy hair of non-Black people in the way that it grows—I will delve more into this later in the book.

So, the afro is not a hair *style*—it is a natural hair form. There is also the societal experience of having Afro hair that is unique to Black people and demands a far more delineated and detailed definition of Afro hair.

As someone with Afro hair, how we speak about it and how it is represented and understood is of huge importance to me. When having conversations about topics denoting wider Black culture and history, it is imperative that Black people are leading the conversation and that we are having the conversation in the first place. As we will see over the course of this book, the Afro is a natural hair form that has been pulled in many different directions (no pun intended), and one that has been at the centre of contemporary conversation for quite some time, yet the depth and rich societal context behind it is something that often gets misconstrued, simplified and often disrespected. This is why I am so passionate about the *A Quick Ting On* series—it provides space to explore these topics pertaining to Black culture in a free and unlimited way. Now, onto the topic in question: hair.

My experiences with my hair have shaped me into the person that I am today, and it has been far from a smooth ride. When I was younger, I wished that I could have the long straight hair of my white friends. As a child, I also wished that my mother had allowed me to use chemical products to alter my hair texture like some of my other Black friends did. I've felt frustration with my hair, I have grown tired of attempting to manage and care for my hair, I've had people stare at and touch my hair as if I'm an animal at the zoo and there were times where I would look at my hair in the mirror and not see its beauty. My hair and I have gone through it all. Today, I have learnt to own my hair, I have grown to love my hair and feel confident in whatever way I choose to wear it.

If you are reading this and thinking, "what is the big fuss? It's just hair". Well, as I write this book, Black children are still being suspended from schools because their naturally Afro hair is seen as 'breaching uniform policy'. Black people are still being told that their Afro hair is unprofessional and shouldn't be sported in the workplace and somewhere, right now there is a Black girl with her beautiful afro out and an unwelcome hand grabbing it unprovoked.

But there is hope. The natural hair movements, both in the 1960s and in more recent years, have helped defy the ideals that society places on Black women. Whether this movement is truly inclusive is a different question that we will explore later, but its message is powerful. The rise of social media has given Black women a platform to connect, share their hair experiences, obtain guidance and showcase beautiful styles. Black women in Britain hold a huge amount of economic power; the Black hair care industry is worth an estimated £88 million and Black women spend at least three times more on their hair than white women.[1] In America, the Black hair care industry is worth over $2 billion. Most large manufacturers of hair products in the West have overlooked Black hair for a long time, by offering products that didn't work well on Afro-textured hair, or not offering any appropriate products at all. The number of independent Black-owned businesses making healthy products for Afro hair both in the UK and stateside is increasing. There's an opportunity for them to dominate the market as more and more mainstream products are being exposed as damaging and unsatisfactory for Afro hair.

This book is expansive in the topics it explores, and this was an intentional decision between me and my editor. The afro as a subject matter is wide ranging and multi-dimensional. We felt that it was important to explore it from its political and economical angle, its scientific angle and of course through the lens of the ever so important experiences of Black women. For this book, I conducted a survey with over 350 Black women. The aim of this research was to obtain anecdotal evidence about the experiences faced by Black British women in relation to their hair, and their views of various hair related topics.

I hope this book is a useful resource for Black women and girls, one that helps them feel supported in their own hair journeys. I want Black women to read this book and feel represented—we've all had our own unique experiences and it's important that these stories are told. For people who may not know much about this topic, I hope you will learn something new and deepen your understanding of Afro hair.

A Quick Ting On: The Black Girl Afro will debunk some hair myths and teach you some new hair tricks. It will also explore the history and depth of Afro hair, highlighting topics such as the science of Afro hair, all the way to how the afro is represented and understood in society today. This book, at times, may make you laugh, cry and smile. It was a labour of love and I am so pleased to finally be able to share it with you.

1

ME, MYSELF AND MY AFRO

It's 1998. I am sitting on the living room floor in front of the TV, in-between my mum's legs, watching *The Lion King* on video tape. My mum holds a thick-toothed comb and scores it across my scalp. She parts my hair into six equal sections. Taking the first section, she combs through my hair, starting from the ends and slowly making her way towards my roots. My tight curls, like always, protest against my mother's motion. She rakes through them more firmly. I let out a sharp inhale and rub my hand on my scalp, whilst trying to wiggle my way out from the clasp of her legs. She nudges my hand away with the comb and calmly says, 'don't move or it will hurt even more'. I know this, but I can't help but flinch and squirm as she weaves my hair into thick plaits. She blows gently on my scalp. I'm not sure if it helps, but it gives me some comfort.

Experiences like this form some of my earliest childhood memories. My daily routine as a child involved my mum cleaning, detangling and neatly styling my hair each morning to ensure that I was ready for school. By the time my mum would collect me at the end of the day, she could barely recognise the immaculate hairstyle that once was. With the loose stray hairs and unravelled plaits all over the place, my mother was convinced that I spent my days wrestling rather than sitting in lessons. Our evenings would consist of freeing my hair of the braids and letting my hair loose. It wouldn't be long before my mum would instruct me to sit down so that she could comb the tangles out of my thick hair—it was a moment I dreaded for many years. It was a painful ordeal that often left me on the verge of tears. To make me feel better, my mum would massage my scalp with oils whilst we watched TV. Now, I look back on these memories with nostalgia. Getting my hair done provided me with deeply intimate moments with my mother. Even though I didn't always enjoy it, I generally felt soothed when she was tending to my hair. There was something incredibly reassuring about being in her grasp, her hands working fervently through my scalp. It felt safe. It felt like home.

I loved Disney films as a child and was particularly fond of the character of Pocahontas, not just because of her songs (although she did have some classics... give Pocahontas her Grammys right now!). My draw towards Pocahontas was because of her brown skin. Here was a character who looked more like me than any other character I had ever seen. Even so, if you have seen me and Pocahontas, you will know how wildly different we are, but she was all I had. She was the character that I always wanted to dress up as for World Book Day or any other event that required a fancy dress costume. I loved her long waist-length hair; it wasn't the usual blonde or mouse-brown hair on all the other Disney princesses—it was black like mine. However, there was one discrepancy. Her hair was dead straight. There seemed to be no place for curly hair in Disney films. As a result, I found myself yearning for Pocahontas's straight hair. In front of the mirror, I would hold some of my tight curls and slowly pull, stretching them out until they were almost straight. Eventually, I would let go of my hair and watch it spring back into its usual zigzag shape. I would stay staring at my afro in the mirror, envisioning what it would be like to have long, flowing, straight hair. This childhood ritual is one that many Black women could probably relate to at one stage in their lives.

Interestingly, the desire to have straight hair was not motivated by how I was viewed by others, but more by how I wanted to see myself. Over the course of my life, I have felt many emotions towards and about my hair, from indifference to curiosity, which would later become embarrassment followed by hatred. Today, I only feel love and acceptance towards my hair, which is a far cry from the young Zainab who used to pull at her curls hoping they would magically straighten.

Family played a huge role in how I understood and saw my hair as a child. My first memory of other people's perceptions of my hair relates to one of my Ghanaian aunts. She was actually my late father's cousin, but I referred to her as my auntie, as is typically done in African homes. My dad passed away before I was old enough to start school, and it was this auntie who would look after me whilst my mum was at work. Whenever I would interact with her, she would greet me with a big hug and say, 'give me some of your hair, you have enough for me too!' This may seem like a trivial interaction, but it would be my auntie's positive assertions that sparked my initial curiosity about my hair. Her comments would make me feel special and proud of my hair. Unbeknownst to my auntie or myself at the time, she set an important foundation in my hair journey, one that I would at times stray from but would eventually come back to.

Being the youngest out of three, my older sisters, Zahra and Bishara, were girls I looked up to. Being respectively six and four years older than me, I witnessed them starting secondary school, entering their teenage years and discovering themselves whilst I was still a child. I would watch them experimenting with their hair at a time when I was too young to manage my own. We'd go to the local Black hair shop with my mum and scour the aisles like children in a sweetshop. These shops had it all—colourful shampoos, conditioners, moisturisers, wigs, combs, make-up, jewellery, perfumes and creams!

Under my mum's instructions, we would grab the necessary items from the shelves and place them into our basket before rushing home to review our inventory. This hair shopping routine was not something exclusive to us; many Black girls and women have undergone and continue to undergo this sacred pilgrimage. As per the routine, once we had arrived home, we would sit eagerly in our bedroom and I would get to observe my sisters lay out their new brushes, thick and thin-toothed combs, beads, rubber bands and hair gels. It was the stuff of beautifying dreams. My sisters would trace their hands over colourful packet after colourful packet, and eventually pick up the gel container and rip open a bag full of beads. Then the fun part would begin—my sisters would begin plaiting, twisting, tying or slicking their hair into intricate styles. I would stare in awe. The versatility of Black hair, even then, blew me away and I couldn't wait until I could learn to style my own.

I was about eight years old when my sisters first discovered hair relaxer, a chemical product that alters your hair to make it straight. Although my mum disapproved of their use of hair relaxer, it was more important to her that my siblings had the freedom to experiment with their hair. Those of you who have used or come across hair relaxers before will understand what I mean when I say that the smell of that product is truly unforgettable! For those of you who haven't smelt the product, it is something that exudes a pungent and suffocating stench, one that takes me straight back to watching my sisters lather that thick white cream onto their hair. Once the cream's burning became almost unbearable, my sisters would rush to the bathroom to wash out the chemical and observe the result.

The outcome was the transformation of their tight curls into soft, straight strands. This was the first time I saw Afro hair suddenly become straight—just like Pocahontas's hair! As a child, this was the stuff of magic. I was fascinated at how Black hair, which was so curly by nature, could become so straight.

Once I had entered my teenage years, my ideals surrounding Black hair were almost solely influenced by societal standards of beauty, which sadly meant that Afro-textured hair was not something that I looked upon favourably. It was also around this time that my sisters realised the negative effects of chemical relaxers on their hair and stopped using it. As a result, my family forbade me from ever relaxing my hair. At the time, I was devastated—my kinky, fuzzy hair wasn't cool, and my teenage years were meant to be my time to experiment with my hair. Upon reflection, I'm grateful for my family's collective decision to protect my hair.

So there I was: a short, nerdy, Black teenager with Afro hair, going to school in the middle-class suburbs. You know where this is going, right?

My school days consisted of students shoving their hands into my hair to feel how 'fluffy' it was. The nicer kids would give my hair a squeeze or bury their face in it whilst 'complimenting' me by describing my hair as something relatively inoffensive, such as a cloud or pillow. The meaner kids would make nasty comments and throw bits of paper or stick pencils in my hair. I vividly recall wearing my hair in two bunches ('Afro puffs') and hearing a boy in my class announce that, 'Zainab has gorilla testicles on her head', and as you can imagine, the class erupted in a loud chorus of laughter, because that is just what teenagers do. I was 14 at the time. I rolled my eyes and shrugged the comment off as though I didn't care, but deep down I was filled with shame and embarrassment.

With Black people my age, it wasn't so straightforward either. Even amongst my own community, I still felt like an outsider, in part, because so many of my peers wore extensions and relaxed their hair. As the years would go by, I began to receive comments from Black people (friends and strangers alike), which added to the complex feelings I already felt towards my hair:

'I wish I had hair like yours, mine doesn't grow like that.'

'If you relaxed your hair, it would look so nice.'

'Your hair is so nice for a Black girl—where are you from?'

Despite Afro hair still being unpopular at the time, I was constantly reminded by those from my community that I was lucky or special for having hair like mine. So, I felt othered almost everywhere.

Black women relaxing their hair is like a rite of passage, but this is something that I'd never experienced. It played a role in oddly making me feel isolated when discussing hair and beauty with other Black women in my life. Of all the comments I would hear from the gorgeous Black girls who sported weaves or relaxed their hair, it was the comment of, 'your hair would be so pretty if it was straight' that made me feel that my natural curls made me unattractive.

When evaluating the common emotions I felt towards or about my hair growing up, guilt was always a regular one. Interestingly, the way in which guilt cropped up in relation to my hair was multidimensional. For example, there was *this* question that I would get that made me cower: 'what did you do to make your hair look like that?' I would usually mumble something that explained that this was simply the natural state of my hair, to which I would be met with a disappointing stare or an unimpressed sigh. I had wished that I could give an answer that people would find useful or interesting, but I never could. Then there was the whole hair-touching fiasco that any girl with an Afro can relate to. This interaction also invited pangs of guilt, embarrassment and, at times, frustration. The guilt surfaced when I would decline people's requests to touch my hair, particularly those who were very polite about it. I would often resign to allowing the polite requestees to touch my hair to avoid potentially upsetting them by saying no.

DJ, CUE SOLANGE KNOWLES' 'DON'T TOUCH MY HAIR'

When it comes to chronic afro touchers, there are usually two types: 1)Those who are considerate and ask for my consent beforehand, which is appreciated, I guess, though it still brings forward an uncomfortable and awkward situation, which I would rather not deal with, and, 2)Those who go straight for a grab or pet of the afro without asking, which, as you can imagine, is highly frustrating and quite dehumanising.

My university experience was a truly testing period when it

came to my hair. Let me tell you, attending a predominantly white university when you have an afro is an experience that will stay with you! In part, this is because university is a place where young people, drugs and alcohol meet in abundance and not to forget, many attendees do not come from big, diverse cities, so seeing an afro in person was a new experience for many white students.

Before I delve into my university experience, I would like to shout out all the drunk white girls from the University of Bristol whom I met whilst partying in clubs, who gushed over my hair whilst complaining that they wished they had a curly afro like mine because it has so much volume, or asking whether I think their hair would look nice if it was braided because they really wanted to get canerows when they went on holiday. It was an overwhelming amount of information to unpack in the middle of the ladies toilets on a Monday night, but hey, that's student life for you.

Personally, these types of interaction didn't particularly bother me—I actually found them amusing, tolerable and at times a little flattering. The people I had absolutely no patience for, however, were the students (usually male) who used my hair as the butt of their jokes and carelessly messed with it for their own entertainment. Once, I had my hair braided and was walking back to my flat after a long day of revision, and a group of white boys ran past me shouting, 'love your shitlocks, babe!' Imagine being so ignorant that you can't even insult me correctly. Sir, these are BRAIDS, not locks. Tragic.

One night, I was so sick of my hair being mocked and touched that when a guy came up from behind me in a bar and buried his hands into my perfectly shaped afro, I turned around to face him and ran my hand through his neatly gelled hair to ruffle it up. He immediately shoved me and told me not to touch him because I had ruined his hair. Therein lies the hypocrisy of it all—people understand that invasion of privacy is unacceptable if it happens to them, but my afro was the exception—it was everyone's property.

Another facet of the guilt I held as a Black girl with an afro was the conspicuous nature of my hair. As strange as it may sound, I was constantly concerned that my hair was in the way of others. There is a heightened sense of self-awareness that comes with having Afro hair in public. Whether it is at the cinema, theatre, university lecture or work conference, the feeling is always there.

As a result, I would automatically sit at the back of rooms or at the end of a row of seats. This burden was ingrained in me due to the number of comments that people made about my hair.

'Excuse me, I can't see anything because of your hair.'

'Your hair is in the way, love.'

'Do you mind moving to the back?'

One particular space that invited perhaps the most height-ened sense of self-consciousness about my hair was public transport. Public transport in London is chaotic at the best of times, and during rush hour it is truly the devil's playground. I've found myself stuck underneath armpits, pushed against chests, and people have also found their faces stuck in my hair. Usually, when the underground was particularly busy, in an attempt to keep my hair out of anyone's way, I would stay as close to the train doors as possible until, one day, the doors closed ON my hair. Awful, right?

Typically, if something gets caught between the tube doors, the train is able to detect it and the doors will reopen until the obstruction is removed. Unfortunately for me, my hair was not thick enough for the tube doors to detect that it was there, but it also wasn't thin enough to fall out from between the doors. As a result, I was stuck there with the tube hurtling through the tunnel with my hair trapped in the doors. If I had softer, straighter hair, I'm sure my hair would have slipped right through, but as a woman with an afro, even public transport can oppress you!

So, in my long list of awkward afro chronicles, having my hair stuck in the tube doors is definitely in my Top 5. The embarrassing and slightly traumatic ordeal did, however, come with an important lesson, one that as a young adult, I take everywhere. That is, do not hide, tame, or conceal your afro for other people because if you do, you will end up getting your hair dragged in the doors of a dirty train along the Piccadilly line.

Nowadays, I relish the fact that I have big hair when I'm commuting to work. My hair acts as my very own shield, protecting me from the horrors of the London underground. My fellow commuters, in true polite British fashion, try their best to, quite literally, stay out of my hair. This means I always have a small amount of space around me, which is much appreciated.

It saddens me to think that I once felt hatred towards my hair. Any feelings I've had towards my hair, good and bad, have never started and ended solely with my hair. They were inexplicably linked to how I viewed my own Blackness at the time.

Growing up in the '90s and 2000s, I became aware that being dark-skinned was socially undesirable. In popular culture, 'beautiful' women were typically white or of a lighter skin tone. On top of this, the few figures of Black beauty who were celebrated such as Naomi Campbell, Beyonce and Tyra Banks, often sported long, straight or wavy hair. Hair like mine didn't make it into the movies, music videos and on the catwalk. So, of course, as a child, all I could assume was that my hair was ugly.

For someone who hates her hair so much, you may be wondering when I finally began altering my hair to *fit in*. Well, this part of my hair story happened in my teen years when I was FINALLY allowed to use hair straighteners. As a Black girl, it takes a while to figure out how to care for your hair and as a teenager I hadn't the slightest idea what I was doing. Information on how to look after Black hair wasn't as readily available as it is today, so I did my best with the limited tools and information I had.

So, I broke my hair straightener virginity, and my teen years were filled with me ironing out my kinks and curls until my hair was unrecognisable. I loved it! My hair was finally flowing down my back rather than sticking out in all directions. I now fitted in. I had *normal*, soft, straight hair just like the other girls in school, and no one could tease me about my big poofy afro anymore.

A young Zainab knew nothing about heat damage, but she sure would learn. When I got to university, my hair was shorter, thinner and unhealthy. I would learn that this destruction was due to the excessive heat from the hair straighteners. I was devastated—having straight hair made me feel more accepted, more comfortable and more beautiful. Now, not only was it shorter, but I had also sacrificed the health of my hair. I knew that if I kept this up, I could end up permanently damaging my hair. So, reluctantly, I began to ebb and flow between having my hair natural and straightening it. Eventually I would wear protective styles and develop a hair care routine that brought my hair back to health again.

University, for me, was a time to become reacquainted with a newer, slightly more mature Zainab. I took time to make new friends and invest in the activities I was passionate about. I wanted to be unapologetically myself and encourage others to do the same. All of this played a part in me gaining a new-found confidence and learning to love my hair and Blackness. I began owning the things that made me unique, especially my afro.

As time went on, I found that the more I owned my hair, the more it became an integral part of me, and the more I celebrated it, the more others seemed to celebrate it too.

My hair priority is now to have healthy, happy hair that I love, irrespective of the thoughts of others. The versatility of my afro is now something I am proud of, and it is something that makes me feel beautiful. So, whilst I no longer sit in-between my mum's legs as she caringly tends to my hair, I have recreated that calm, safe feeling for myself whenever I give my hair the love it deserves.

2

HAIR STORY:
THE HISTORY OF THE AFRO

Black hair as a subject is a central part of Black history. When we assess and explore such a subject, we find it provides us with valuable and important information about Black people and culture from a global perspective. Therefore, to understand the context of Black hair in the contemporary age, we must first look at the history of Black hair.

AFRICA

In many African cultures, hair holds significant societal meanings. From the start of most traceable African civilizations, hair has long been a marker of things such as class, financial status, marital status and ethnicity. In some African cultures, if a woman had untidy or unkempt hair, it indicated that she was going through a difficult period in life. Hair being symbolic of life stages in Africa even extends to the mourning process, where in some African cultures, it is common for recently widowed women to shave their hair as part of a grieving ritual. So as you can tell, when it comes to Africa, hair was and is *literally* life.

In West African communities, Kuramo men, who are a group native to Nigeria, were recognised by their partially shaved hairstyle.[1] The Wolof people of Senegal were known for styling their hair elaborately with different hairstyles being indicative of different life experiences. For example, a Wolof man would wear a particular braided style to indicate that he was about to go to war and was preparing for death.[2]

For the Maasai tribe of Kenya and Tanzania in East Africa,[3] shaving one's hair represents a new start and is often a symbol of entering adulthood. When young Masai men become warriors, they grow their hair and style it into intricate small braids using ochre, a natural clay that gives the hair an orange colour when applied.

Across the African continent hair is believed to be sacred and to bear a spiritual connection to those it belongs to, so much so, that, in some African countries, it is believed that a strand of hair is all that is needed to perform witchcraft on a person.[4]

SLAVERY

When European people travelled to the continent of Africa in the 1400s, they documented their fascination with the intricate hairstyles they observed as well as learning about how such styles related to identity and status.[5]

Throughout the 1500s, Britain and other European countries formed colonies across Africa and wanted human labour for the mass production of crops on those lands. The Europeans transported Africans from West Africa to plantations in America and the Caribbean in the early 1600s. This marked the start of the Transatlantic slave trade and the beginning of hundreds of years of oppression and exploitation of African people.

One of the first acts physically enforced onto the enslaved African people by the Europeans was the cutting of all of their hair. It is generally understood that this was done, in part, for sanitary reasons.[6] However, for enslaved Africans, the impact of such an action was far deeper. Part of the justification of slavery was that African people were inferior and sub-human. This, alongside the fact that hair had and continues to hold importance across the continent, meant that Europeans shaving the heads of enslaved Africans worked to literally strip them of their identity and traditions, symbolically removing their cultural ties to Africa. Enslaved people were left with no way to care for their hair, which meant their hair matted, becoming unkempt and uncared for.

When we look at enslaved African women in particular, the removal of their hair occurred for another darker reason. There were many cases where white women were jealous of the fact that slave masters would rape enslaved women and force them to be their mistresses. In retaliation, white women would shave the heads of enslaved women in an attempt to remove their femininity and make them less attractive to the slave masters.

During this time, it is believed that African people used their hair as a means of survival. Knowing that they were about to be enslaved and would have access to little food when being taken to America and the Caribbean, African people would hide rice grains and seeds in their scalp,[7] disguising them using cornrow (or canerow) braiding styles. Although not documented widely, it is thought that this was a key contributing factor to the growth of the rice industry in America and the Caribbean. European slave masters learnt how to grow rice from the enslaved people and began to sell it on a wider scale.

Hair also became a crucial method for communicating hidden messages to fellow slaves without alerting slave masters. For example in Colombia, the braiding of hair was used to communicate possible escape routes.[8] More specifically, when enslaved Afro-Colombian women were ready to escape, they would wear a braided style known as 'departes'.[9]

In 1786, the Tignon law was created in Louisiana, which legally banned Black women from wearing their hair out in public. The purpose of this was to keep the enslaved and recently freed Black population under control—to remove their identity and uniqueness. Black women were required to cover their hair at all times with a material called a 'tignon'. This ultimately backfired on the lawmakers since Black women responded to this by wearing colourful and gorgeously put together head wraps, making them even more attractive to admirers of the opposite sex.[10]

After centuries of oppression and countless attempts of having an identity stripped away, it is no surprise that the journey to accepting and celebrating one's Blackness and natural hair is not always a smooth one.

The Transatlantic slave trade would techincally end in 1865, and the slave trade in the Caribbean would techincally end in 1834.[11] I say 'technically' because 'freed' Black people still suffered gravely after these slave trades were officiated as over.

There was one key difference between slavery ending in America and in the Caribbean. In America, once enslaved people were freed, they were released into a world where they had to live alongside white people, which was not the case for those who remained in the Caribbean. White Americans who were used to seeing Black people as inferior were forced to accept that these people were now 'free.' Black people having to assimilate into a society where their physical essence was seen as inferior and unattractive was an extremely challenging experience. Despite their best efforts, existing in a world where white skin and straight hair rendered you more human and deserving of economic opportunities, at times, proved impossible.

INVENTIONS

In 1870s France, Francois Marcel Grateau invented a hair straightening tool known as the hot comb.[12] Using iron rods heated over a fire, he created an S-shaped hairstyle named the Marcel Wave, which became extremely popular amongst white women in France and gave Marcel huge amounts of success. Decades later, the hot comb would become a must-have accessory amongst Black women when African-American entrepreneur, Madame CJ Walker, created her own version of the hair styling tool.[13] Hot combs have evolved over the years into curling tongs and flat irons that are incredibly popular amongst all women today.

At the start of 1910, an African-American man called Garrett Augustus Morgan accidentally created a liquid that smoothed out the texture of wool cloth,[14] whilst trying to create a product to lubricate parts of sewing machines. He then tested this substance on a dog, followed by himself, and realised that he had created a product that could straighten hair. Yes, you guessed it... chemical hair relaxers were born! At a time where natural Black hair was stopping African-American people from progressing, Morgan's invention (which he called Hair Refining Cream) provided a solution that enabled both men and women to straighten their hair and assimilate slightly more easily into American society.

In the 1900s, African-American entrepreneur and inventor

Annie Turnbo Malone began experimenting with products that could help with baldness and hair breakage.[15] Malone set up The Poro Company in 1900 to sell her product, the Wonderful Hair Grower, and recruited other Black women who were able to earn a commission from the products they sold.[16] Malone used her success to set up the first US training school for African-American hairstyling, as well as donating to several causes to support Black people.

Madame CJ Walker also wanted to find a solution to repair damaged hair. She was employed by Malone for a short period before deciding to launch her own range of products in 1905. Madame CJ Walker is documented as the first self-made female millionaire in America. Similar to Malone, she donated to multiple charities that supported the African-American community.

In the UK, Len Dyke, Dudley Dryden and Tony Wade would embark on a similar journey of Black hair entrepreneurship in the mid-1960s. Dyke and Dudley opened up their travel agency and record distribution company called Dyke & Dryden Ltd.[17] Soon after, Wade would join them as a director, and they would decide to enter the Black hair and beauty business. They would go on to carve out a beauty and hair empire, with their company becoming the face of the industry in the UK.[18] The Dyke & Dryden Ltd company would become the first Black multi-million-pound business in Britain.

In 1954, African-American entrepreneur George Johnson started the company Johnson Products with his wife Joan Johnson. They launched Ultra Wave, a hair relaxer for Black men, followed by Ultra Sheen, which was a relaxer targeted at Black women. The product was marketed as a more efficient way to achieve straight hair over tools such as the hot comb. Johnson's business was a huge success and similar to the entrepreneurs before him, he used his profits to invest back into the Black community.[19] Interestingly, Johnson Products would become the main sponsor for the infamous African-American show *Soul Train*.

The thriving Black hair market would eventually catch the attention of huge hair conglomerates and manufacturers. Giant companies such as Revlon began offering to purchase small Black-owned hair businesses, including offering to acquire Johnson Products for $100million in 1970, a sale that never went through.[20] By 1985, this new business tactic would lead to Revlon having lead sales in hair relaxers.[21]

Although Malone, Walker and Johnson's success was a huge benefit to Black communities, their businesses perpetuated the idea that Black hair had to be altered and straightened to be acceptable.

As the Black Power movement took off, Black people began rejecting European standards of beauty. This would result in the decline of hair straightening products between the 1950s and 1970s. With sales rapidly decreasing and big manufacturers taking over, existing Black businesses who specialised in hair straightening products saw themselves in a predicament. Many hairstylists and companies went out of business as a result, but George E. Johnson expanded the Ultra Wave and Ultra Sheen ranges to cater to natural hair too,[22] successfully staying relevant in a changing US market. In the UK, Dyke & Dryden Ltd expanded their offering and launched the afro comb in the UK,[23] which was a symbol of Black pride as well as a necessary tool to maintain the perfect 'fro.

THE BLACK POWER MOVEMENTS

The Black Power movements in the US and UK throughout the '60s were a direct challenge to the way that Black people were treated and seen within society. The movement, in turn, birthed powerful expressions of art, protest, business, creativity and ultimately change, all in the spirit of combatting systemic racism and celebrating Blackness. Part of this meant that many Black people made the conscious decision to reject European ideals of beauty and accept what was understood as 'Black Beauty'. This wave of Black consciousness led a substantial amount of the Black population in the US and UK to embrace and proudly sport their natural hair. Thus, the first wave of the natural hair movement began.

The afro, for many, became a political symbol, an act of Black defiance and resistance. For some, namely those who were not in favour of the movement, it was seen as a weapon and a threat. Some of the most iconic images from this period are Black people, such as Angela Davis, with their fists raised high, head to toe in black leather, sporting their perfectly shaped afros in all their glory. Wearing your afro back then was a middle finger to white supremacy. During this period, well known sayings from activists regarding the importance of wearing Afro hair with pride were popular, namely Marcus Garvey's infamous saying, 'don't remove the kinks from your hair, remove them from your brain!'

As the Black Power movement started to die down in the early 1970s, natural Afro hair became more popular and normalised, ultimately losing its association with the political movement. With the peak of the funk music scene in the '70s and '80s, the popularity of the afro as a stylish hairstyle became more commonplace. Around this time, the fashion industry began adopting this look, which played a hand in Afro hair and braiding styles becoming a cool new trend.

Despite the natural hair movement, the need to achieve the 'straight look' was not fully eradicated. The demand for relaxers, hot combs and flat irons was still high and the market of artificial hair, namely wigs, weaves and extensions, would take off in the 1980s,[24] giving Black women an alternative way to style their hair whilst avoiding chemical and heat damage.

As we entered the new millennium, society became reliant on a global computer network also known as 'the internet'. The internet changed every facet of how we consume and share information. This had a huge effect on the world of Black hair. The rise of social media in the 2000s birthed the second wave of the natural hair movement. This was the result of several factors: increased access to information via the web, easily discoverable people and content through social media and the increase of vlogger culture. Interestingly, society's reliance on social media also heralded a number of other movements that we will explore in a later chapter, of which hair was a subset of, namely, body positivity, sustainability and wellbeing.

This present natural hair movement, which I would say is still occuring as I write this book, is not necessarily as political as the first natural hair movement, and I would say, this most recent wave feels as though it has potential to be more long-lasting, in part, because much of it is rooted in concerns for the health of hair rather than just the aesthetic or its political implications.

3

THE POLITICS OF
AFRO HAIR

Whether the discussion is about the natural hair movement, western beauty ideals or the appropriation of Black hair, a common rebuttal to all of these talking points is that 'it's just hair'. When talking to non-Black people about the fact that I was writing this book about hair, I was often asked why it was just about Black women and why specifically Afro hair. It wasn't until I explained some of my own experiences that the need for such a book was understood. The reality is that for Black people, hair is rarely JUST hair.

It wasn't just hair when in 2014, British blogger and model Simone Powderly was told to change her hairstyle (braids) to secure a job she had interviewed for with a luxury recruitment agency, and when she refused, she was not offered the role. It wasn't just hair when in 2016, Google came under fire because their image search results for 'unprofessional hairstyles for work' consisted almost entirely of Black women with Afro hair, whilst on the contrary, 'professional hairstyles for work' displayed pictures exclusively of white women. It wasn't just hair when that same year, teenage students of Pretoria High School in South Africa had to protest because they weren't allowed to wear their natural hair at school. It wasn't just hair when in 2020, 18-year-old Ruby Williams had to take legal action against her school after she was sent home several times because teachers claimed her Afro hair was against uniform policy.

In order to delve into the experiences, challenges, and nuances surrounding Black women's hair, *A Quick Ting On* creator, Mags, suggested I conduct an online survey to hear directly from Black British women. Mags and I sat down at a members' club in central London and decided on what kind of thoughts we felt Black British women would want to express about their hair. The survey was called 'Black British Women and their hair' and more than 350 Black British women completed the survey over 8 weeks. The survey asked them a range of questions about their relationship with their hair, as well as their thoughts on wider topics regarding Black hair. The respondents ranged from teenagers to over 50-year-olds.

Reading through the survey responses made me feel emotional. My aim for this book was not to only include my own experiences—it was important that I captured the voices and perspectives of as many Black women as possible. Reading the stories of these people whom I didn't even know was incredibly validating. Not all survey participants had the same experiences; however, one thing that remained consistent was that participants often had deeply personal and complex hair journeys.

WHEN IT COMES TO YOUR RELATIONSHIP WITH YOUR HAIR, WHICH STATEMENT APPLIES TO YOU THE MOST?

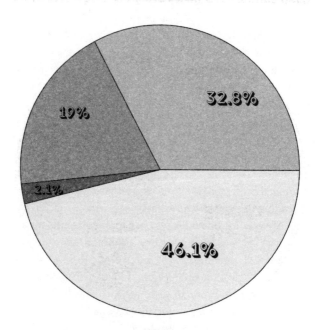

- I PREVIOUSLY HAD SOME ISSUES/STRUGGLES WITH MY HAIR BUT I HAVE OVERCOME THEM AND NOW LOVE IT

- I HAVE HAD A DIFFICULT JOURNEY WITH MY HAIR AND AM STILL IN THE PROCESS OF LEARNING TO LOVE IT

- MY JOURNEY HAS BEEN MAINLY POSITIVE AND I HAVE NEVER REALLY HAD ANY ISSUES WITH MY HAIR

- MY JOURNEY HAS BEEN MAINLY NEGATIVE AND I DON'T THINK I'LL EVER BE ABLE TO FULLY LOVE MY HAIR

PLEASE RATE THE FOLLOWING STATEMENT: 'BLACK WOMEN'S HAIR IS A POLITICAL STATEMENT—NO MATTER HOW THEY WEAR IT.'

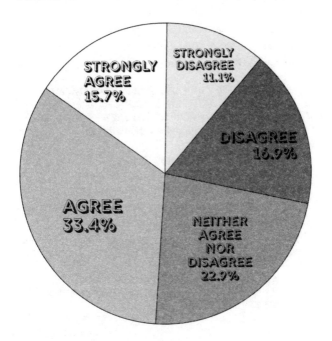

STRONGLY DISAGREE 11.1%

DISAGREE 16.9%

STRONGLY AGREE 15.7%

AGREE 33.4%

NEITHER AGREE NOR DISAGREE 22.9%

When respondents were asked to describe their relationship with their hair, the results were mixed. The most common option (selected by 46.1% of respondents) was: 'I previously had some issues/struggles with my hair but I have overcome them and now I love it', which is quite a positive response and would certainly be the one I would have chosen had I had done the survey. However, it highlights the point made earlier that a Black woman's hair journey is very rarely smooth sailing, but more a gradual process of acceptance and self-love.

This response was followed by 32.8% of respondents expressing: 'I have had a difficult journey with my hair and am still in the process of learning to love it'. This indicates that a substantial amount Black women are faced with challenges when it comes to their hair, but the positive side is that many of them can overcome these obstacles, or at least envision doing so. Only 18% of respondents chose the statement: 'My

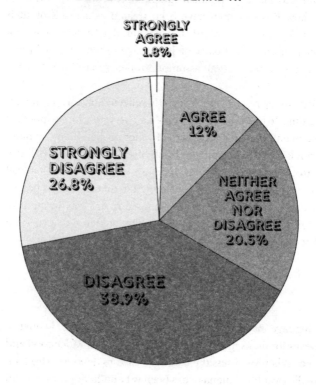

PLEASE RATE THE FOLLOWING STATEMENT:
'THE WAYS BLACK WOMEN WEAR THEIR HAIR THESE DAYS ARE JUST DIFFERENT STYLES—THERE IS NO DEEPER MEANING BEHIND IT.'

STRONGLY AGREE
1.8%

AGREE
12%

NEITHER AGREE NOR DISAGREE
20.5%

STRONGLY DISAGREE
26.8%

DISAGREE
38.9%

journey has been mainly positive and I have never really had any issues with my hair', which to me was not surprising at all.

When presented with the statement: 'Black women's hair is a political statement—no matter how they wear it', half of the respondents answered 'Agree or Strongly Agree', with 22% selecting 'Neither agree nor disagree'.

For the statement: 'The ways Black women wear their hair these days are just different styles—there is no deeper meaning behind it', two-thirds responded with 'Disagree or Strongly Disagree'. Most of the respondents agreed that Black women's hair was indeed a political statement that directly correlates to how Black women have been treated as a result of their hair. As we have previously touched on, Black women have not been afforded the luxury of being able to style their hair any way they want, without assumptions being made about them.

One survey respondent succinctly reflected on this sentiment, writing: 'I think Black women's hair is very often a political statement, but only in the eyes of other people. In my opinion, I think it's rarely the intention of Black women to be political with their hair, usually, they are just wearing styles they like! But it's viewed by others as being a statement. I've had people give me the Black power fist for having my hair in an afro, when the reality was, I just couldn't be bothered to style it up that day.'

'THAT GOOD HAIR': COLOURISM AND TEXTURISM

Language gives us a vehicle to express culture. It is often a means for us, as individuals and groups, to be understood and seen. When we assess the language used to describe Afro hair, we discover that language has been yet another oppressive tool working against it.

Words commonly used to describe Afro hair such as nappy, frizzy, unruly and bushy have negative connotations, implying that Afro hair is fundamentally not good. The use of these words shape the way that young Black children view their hair and can result in lower self-esteem when comparing their hair to their white peers.

There is an urgent need to *untangle* the language of Afro hair (pun intended). If you are Black, it is likely that you have heard the term 'good hair'. Chris Rock made a hit documentary about it, Beyoncé even referred to her husband's mistress as 'Becky with the good hair' in her song 'Sorry'—yes, that's right, the woman who Jay-Z allegedly cheated with had a specific hair type which was a cause for concern!

So, what exactly is 'good hair' and why is it such a problematic phrase? Well, to gain a fundamental understanding of that, we have to leave Beyoncé's *Formation* album (sorry Bey) and go back in time, first to the 1980s, and then back to slavery.

In 1983, activist, author and Pulitzer Prize winner Alice Walker is thought to have coined the term colourism.[1] Colourism is the 'prejudicial or preferential treatment of same-race people based solely on their color.' In a nutshell, colourism is the preference for lighter skin. It is a byproduct of racism and is prevalent in many communities around the world. Whereas racism relates to everyone in a particular racial group, colourism causes a divide between members of the same racial group. From colourism came another '-ism' known as texturism, which is the idea that certain natural hair patterns and hair types are preferred or seen as more desirable than others. More specifically, it is the preference for hair that is looser or softer in pattern and texture than those with coarser or kinkier hair, usually within the same race.

During the South African Apartheid, the Population Registration Act of 1950 required South Africans to be categorised into racial groups. As a person racial make-up was not always apparent, tests were created to establish racial identity. One such test was famously known as the 'pencil test'. This test consisted of a process where a pencil was pushed through an individual's hair and based on the result, the individual would be assigned to a racial group—if the pencil slid through your hair, you were seen as a white person; if the pencil remained in your hair, you were seen as a Black person.[2] For Black people who wanted to identify as biracial or mixed, they would be ordered to shake their head. If the pencil fell out of their hair, they were seen as a mixed-race person, which was understood as more desirable than being fully Black.[3]

During slavery, enslaved women were often raped and subsequently impregnated by their slave masters, giving birth to biracial children who would also be enslaved. Enslaved people with lighter skin were often made to work within the slave masters' houses rather than on the fields and plantations where the darker-skinned slaves worked. It was generally understood that working on the fields was more laborious and difficult than working in the slave master's house. Thus, the lighter-skinned slave was understood to have preferential treatment over the darker-skinned slave. The lighter-skinned slaves were in closer physical proximity to whiteness, namely, due to their looser or softer hair, finer facial features and lighter skin tone. All of this caused divide amongst the enslaved people, and these ideals carried through once the slave trade ended.

Hair, in this context, is a powerful signifier of race. Even in times when someone can pass as a white person due to their complexion and facial features, a kink in their hair may be the only clue to their Black ancestry. Similarly, the closer a person's hair is to caucasian hair, the more likely people are to believe that the individual has white European blood in them. Given that whiteness is often associated with value, success and beauty in the Western world, the closer to whiteness that one could be meant a heightened quality of life for that individual. In this sense, 'good hair' literally equated to a 'good life'. Thus, the modification of natural hair to be straighter or softer was, in actuality, a matter of survival and social mobility.

RACISM

⬇

COLOURISM

⬇

TEXTURISM

Today, these concepts of 'good hair' and 'bad hair' in the wider Black community are still prevalent. The idea that some Black people are born with hair that is naturally **good** (usually those with wavy, looser, softer curls), whereas others are born with hair that is automatically **bad** (usually those with coarser, thicker, kinkier tighter curls that grows upwards), is incredibly damaging and is related to the aftermath of years of racial oppression.

The notion of 'good hair' and 'bad hair' is not an idea exclusive to the Black community. I have lost count of the number of times my white friends have complained about what they call a 'bad hair day' or equally celebrate when they are having a 'good hair day'.

Generally speaking, a good hair day is understood to be a day when your hair looks great and your day also turns out to be great. Thus, a bad hair day is a day where your hair just isn't working for you and it, in turn, colours the experience of your day. An example of a good hair day is a lady who is pleased that her fringe is super straight and flat compared to days when it sticks out in all directions. An example of a bad hair day is a woman wearing her hat for too long, and unfortunately now has hat hair for the rest of the afternoon.

The crucial difference is that when we talk about a 'good hair day' and a 'bad hair day' in this context, they are viewed as temporary states. On the contrary, Black women are told that their hair is either intrinsically good or bad. What does this mean in practice? It means that you have young Black girls growing up to believe that they have permanently undesirable, problematic hair that needs to be 'fixed' or 'corrected'. This sentiment was captured by one of the survey respondents, who wrote: 'When I was a young child my Mum would struggle with my hair saying I had bad hair, my hair wasn't nice, and so I tried all the chemicals from secondary school, curly perm, relaxers, braids...'

HAS ANY OF THE FOLLOWING NEGATIVELY INFLUENCED YOUR RELATIONSHIP WITH YOUR HAIR? (TICK ALL THAT APPLY)

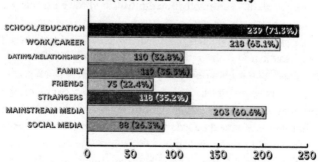

In the 'Black British Women and their hair' survey, when respondents were asked about things that have negatively influenced their relationship with their hair, the top two factors that Black women listed were school/education and work/career. For many of us, these are two environments that we spend a significant proportion of our lives in. The fact that they are the biggest contributors to Black women developing issues with their hair is a tragic reality.

Some respondents offered anecdotal stories of how the school/education environment impacted how they viewed their natural hair.

> 'Going to a predominately white school meant my hair type was seen as different which made it hard to embrace.'

> 'The usual white girls grabbing my hair, touching it, being shocked/appalled/amazed by it.'

> 'Growing up, on TV you would always see girls with long, bone-straight hair and girls at school would show off and sometimes say their hair was better because it was straight. It definitely made me want to have "good" hair that was straight or slightly curly like mixed hair.'

A sad part of the school environment being a frequent space for Black hair discrimination and bullying is that the young girls being picked on will not have the discernment to realise that such ideas are untrue or wrong. Instead, this behaviour works to seep into the impressionable mind of the young, leaving them with the belief that to be normal, successful or beautiful, their hair must be modified.

The anecdotes that were shared in the 'Black British

Women and their hair' survey also shed light on how the home or one's own community can be just as hostile as external spaces. One such anecdote explained, 'My aunties wear mostly wigs and weaves and they weigh their compliments more when I'm wearing a wig or braids instead of having my natural hair out.'

The anecdotes shared in the 'Black British Women and their hair' survey lay bare some of the patterns of hair discrimination amongst children. On the one hand, many report being bullied and picked on by white students due to their natural hair. However, there were also substantial amounts of stories of fellow Black students policing other Black girls' hair and making texturist comments. What does this show? It highlights the colonial paradigm that western environments mimic, as well as showing us how entrenched these views are in the societal psyche.

Of all the respondents' anecdotes, one in particular stuck with me:

> 'I wore my natural hair out (as a punishment for getting in trouble) when I was in year 9. And I wrapped some weave around my bun because I didn't have enough hair to make a bun, and there's a lot of humiliation and shame that comes with Black hair, so when I was asked by my Black classmate whether that hair on my head is real, I, being a child, lied, and that girl pulled the weave off my bun and laughed me down for the hair I was wearing. I actually forgot about this happening—here unpacking some emotional truths. When she was in sixth form, some white girl pulled her wig off in front of everyone, so I am not saying that give and it

> will come back to you (good and bad) but I am
> saying that everything works according to God's
> plan.'

There is a lot to dissect here. Firstly, this respondent's parent or guardian believed that an appropriate way to punish their child was to force them to wear their natural hair. This presumably stemmed from their own anti-Blackness from the experiences they had growing up. Here, we see how texturism and anti-Blackness can be passed down through families who are likely victims of this way of thinking themselves. What this individual went through reinforces the idea that natural hair shouldn't be celebrated or even seen. Instead, it is to be concealed and hidden at all costs like a dirty secret, so much so that this respondent felt as though they had to lie about wearing a weave.

Then, this same girl experiences another Black girl rip her weave off her head. The trauma and violence (both literal and psychological) of such an event cannot be quantified. All actions relating to the girl's hair in this anecdote point to Black hair being despised. This would work to make anyone have a deeply problematic and challenging relationship with their natural hair. It is situations like these that lead to Black women having to actively embark on the journey of learning how to love one's natural hair.

The 'Racism at Work' survey, produced by Pearn Kandola in 2018, reported that 60% of Black people and 42% of Asian people in the UK have experienced racism in the workplace.[4] In my survey, 65.1% of correspondents said that the workplace negatively impacted their relationship with their hair.

Natural hair being seen as unkempt, untidy and untameable means it is seen as the complete antithesis of class and professionalism, particularly in the workplace. Black women in positions of power or success very rarely have their natural hair on display, so much so that a while after the Obama's left office, the previous First Lady, Michelle Obama, wore her natural hair on display and it was the talk of the town. Whilst Obama was celebrated for wearing her hair natural, there was acknowledgement, at least amongst Black women, that this celebration was done knowing that she would have never sported her natural hair whilst in the White House. This is because Obama, like many other Black women, knows what the world understands professionalism to look like and sadly, natural hair isn't part of that ideal.

This is a sentiment I have experienced in my own corporate career journey. When I was applying for banking internships whilst at university, I made a conscious effort to straighten my hair when I had to attend an interview. I did this to make my hair emulate Caucasian hair, because this is what I felt that most people in the workplace would be familiar with. I wanted to prove that I would fit into the workplace, and I didn't believe that my Afro hair would convince interviewers of this.

It would seem that research confirms that my worries were valid. A study conducted and published in the journal of *Social Psychological and Personality Science* in 2020 showed that Black women with natural hairstyles such as afros, braids, cornrows and dreadlocks, were less likely to be successful in the job recruitment process than Black women with straightened hair or white candidates in general.[5]

The term code-switching describes the altering of one's appearance, speech and behaviour in the hope of attaining good service, fair treatment, employment or at times for survival. It is a strategy that has been employed by Black people all over the world. Unsurprisingly, research shows that code-switching happens in environments where problematic or negative perceptions and stereotypes of Black people exist.[6] The workplace is often one of those spaces. Black women styling their hair for work is something that is often subject to code-switching.

When reading through the responses relating to the workplace in the 'Black British Women and their hair' survey, many Black women shared similar experiences about their hair not being accepted or appreciated.

'One time, I wore braids to work and someone said I looked like Whoopi Goldberg.'

'I remember going into work with my natural curls out and a colleague saying "what happened? Bad hair day?" and laughed. I remember feeling so awkward because I tried to explain that this is how my hair grows out of my scalp. They were so used to seeing my hair slicked back in a bun or straightened that they couldn't help but comment or attempt to touch it.'

'Changing my hair in a predominately white workplace garners way more attention and questions than I feel comfortable with so I feel reluctant to change. Also, I've felt some pressure to straighten my hair or wear weaves, which aren't my preference.'

'Had an experience when I first started going natural where another Black female, a work colleague, told me I was making a statement by having my hair natural.'

'When I worked in an office, I was told that I looked more professional when my hair was in braids, and maybe I'd have more opportunities if I "did something" with my hair. When I worked in a food factory, I had to wear braids because they didn't have hair nets that catered to "big" hair. If my hair couldn't fit in their hairnets, then I wasn't allowed to work. I was also bullied by managers and co-workers for having "dread-locks"... Even though they were braids. Sigh.'

'With work, I've often felt like I had to make my hair as flat as possible especially in interviews because I'd worry that it could be the reason why I don't get the job.'

'Every Black girl knows the struggle of deciding how to style your hair before a job interview or the anxiety you feel when you get a new hairstyle and have to debut it at your place of work. The comments and attention make it so daunting.'

Given the COVID-19 pandemic and the rapid increase in people working from home, this may help to change the way that we think about professionalism and appearance in relation to the workplace; only time will tell. However, I won't hold my breath just yet. Something tells me that even the force of a global pandemic cannot shake racial and colonial ideals surrounding Black hair.

THE CASE OF RUBY WILLIAMS

Ruby loved her hair when she was a little girl, although she hated the pain that came with getting her hair done (Black girls will be able to relate to this). Ruby often wore her afro out, however, sometimes she wished that she could have straight Caucasian hair like her mother so she would not have to brush it so much.

In terms of the beginning of our hair journeys, Ruby and I are quite similar. We were both advised by our family not to use chemical relaxers in our hair, so instead, we sought solace in hair straighteners. Ruby's father, Lenny, a Rastafarian man, felt very strongly about avoiding chemicals in her hair, and similarly to me, Ruby's older sisters had experimented with relaxers and warned Ruby not to try them.

Ruby was 11 years old and she had just started secondary school when she began straightening her hair. She quickly became addicted and constantly used hair straighteners for a year until she noticed that the heat damage was preventing her hair from growing. Choosing to give her hair a break, Ruby left her hair to grow in its natural state. She would instead blow dry it so that it would look as long as possible, often wearing it tied up into a single puff at the top of her head.

At 14 years old, Ruby cut off all of her damaged ends, leaving her hair shorter and healthier than before. In October 2016, Ruby walked past her headteacher in the corridor of her school. Noticing her, he said, 'your hair is too big, you're going to need to do something about that.'

Ruby always wore her hair in this way, and there hadn't been any issues before, so her parents didn't think much of it when Ruby told them what happened. However, when Ruby went into school the next day, the headteacher advised her to check the rules about hair on the school website and abide by them, otherwise he would have to send her home. That evening, Ruby and her family went onto the school website and saw a rule that said, 'Afro-style hair including buns must be of reasonable size and length'. They were shocked and confused. When did this rule get introduced? What is 'Afro-style' hair and why didn't this rule apply to other hair types? What is the definition of 'reasonable length'?

This immediately rang alarm bells in Ruby's mother's

mind. Kate, who was a teacher herself, felt that this rule was illegal. She contacted the school and began to seek advice from the Equality Advisory & Support Service (EASS). After these discussions, Kate had found that the rule was potentially discriminatory because it singled out one hair type. School uniform and appearance policies are not statutory; there is only guidance issued by the Department for Education. However, this rule appeared to be in breach of the Equality Act of 2010, which protects people in Britain from workplace discrimination. Ruby decided that she did not want to give in and change her natural hair, knowing that the school was in the wrong. As a result, Ruby was sent home multiple times.

Let's just take a step back for a moment. It's 2016 and a child is being told that her natural hair is not suitable for school unless it is contained and hidden away. Parents are being told their child will be denied an education because they have an afro.

What ensued next was nearly three years of a gruelling battle with the school, with Kate contacting the Local Education Authority, the Equality and Human Rights Commission and their local MP to inform them of the discrimination Ruby was experiencing. Meanwhile, Ruby was still being sent home and was even told by her white, male headteacher to consider using a chemical relaxer to make her hair smaller. Ruby's family decided to enlist legal help and support. To avoid any conflict until the situation was resolved, Ruby went to a hairstylist to have her hair braided, a hairstyle which has its own set of challenges. It's an expensive and time consuming style to maintain and also presents a risk of damage if the hair is braided too tightly.

Throughout this period of time, Ruby and her family felt let down by the systems and structures that were supposedly there to protect and support them. The chair of governors for the school sided with the headteacher and defended the hair policy. Ruby's parents then raised a formal complaint to present the issue in front of a panel—a process that was meant to take six weeks but ended up taking a whole year, and was eventually rejected in November 2017. In January 2018, the EHRC decided to take on and fund Ruby's case. They had already been successful in helping 12-year-old Chikayzea Flanders get compensation and settle his case against his school, who banned dreadlocks and told him that he could only return to school once his locks were cut off.[7]

Despite being contacted multiple times, the school completely ignored court proceedings and did not change their policy. Ruby found this to be an incredibly difficult time at school. Many of the teachers who knew Ruby (some of whom were Black) did not speak up or offer much support at the time, perhaps because their own jobs may have been at risk if they did, or perhaps they sided with the headteacher. A picture of Ruby was hung up in class because she was Star Pupil of the Week, and her headteacher had it taken down because of her hair in the photo. She picked up her school yearbook in January 2018, opened it and saw that the school had chosen to use a photo of her from when she first started the school at 11 years old, rather than her most recent school photo like everyone else. In her Year 7 photo, her hair was straightened and tied back, and in her most recent photo, her natural hair was on display. Nearly two years on from the first incident, Ruby was sent home again in the middle of her GCSE exams because of her hair. After Ruby completed her exams in summer 2018, her time at the school was over because she had secured a place at another college to do her A-levels.

Ruby began her A-levels at her new college and her solicitor applied to the court for a default notice, which the school unsurprisingly ignored. Then, suddenly in the summer of

2019, the school objected to the default notice, got legal representation and wanted a full court case. Ruby and her family prepared for court to see if the judge would reverse the default notice and restart legal proceedings (which could have taken another year or so!). Two days before this was due to start, the school offered her a settlement. After the heartbreaking ordeal they had been put through, an exhausted Ruby accepted the settlement as she didn't want this situation to last any longer and interfere with her A-levels or even university.

After this, the school did not engage the EHRC from October 2019 to March 2020. It wasn't until Ruby and her family went to the press independently to raise awareness on how this experience affected her, that the school began to work with the EHRC to review and rewrite its policy, and ultimately adopted an Equality Statement. The school never publicly apologised or acknowledged any wrongdoing.

I remember Ruby's story hitting social media—Twitter in particular. There was a collective outrage about the way that she was treated, and people rightfully rallied behind her. Ruby's case caused many Black women on social media to speak up and share their own hair experiences at school, which sparked a much needed conversation about discriminatory school policies.

Ruby is now a university student and a qualified make-up artist. She continues to campaign, collaborate widely and speak publicly to raise awareness about Afro hair discrimination internationally. She understands that this experience has shaped her life in many ways but is determined to create positive change from the pain and protect other young people from experiencing what she faced.

Today, work is being done to combat hair discrimination in school and the workplace. The CROWN Act in the US is a piece of legislation that bans discrimination against an individual on the basis of their hair texture or style. As of 2021, 8 US states have signed the CROWN Act into law. This is promising progress. There is no equivalent legislation in the UK, however, an organisation called the Halo Collective, comprised of young Black and mixed-raced individuals from London, has produced a set of anti-hair discrimination principles called the Halo Code. Schools and companies can sign up to the Halo Code and commit to joining the fight against hair discrimination. I am hopeful that this is a small step towards the UK adopting anti-hair discrimination legislation in the future. Only then can we ensure that Black people are no longer disadvantaged as a result of their hair.

Another organisation championing Afro hair and raising awareness of hair discrimination is World Afro Day (WAD). WAD aims to 'promote education and appreciation for the unique position of Afro hair, throughout the world'. Created and founded by Michelle De Leon, WAD takes place on 15th September and was started in 2017 in response to the US federal court ruling in 2016 that effectively stated that it is legal to refuse to hire someone because of their dreadlocks.[8] World Afro Day hosts the annual Big Hair Assembly, where schools across the globe can tune into a live stream focused on celebrating Black hair and equality. WAD also offers resources for schools and teachers to access so that they can deliver lessons to educate pupils on Afro hair.

The 'World Afro Day Hair Equality Report' has been described as the most 'significant' research to date, addressing cross generational bias against Afro hair in UK schools. The survey, supported by researchers at De Montfort University and created by World Afro Day, aims to shed a light on Afro hair bias and hair discrimination in UK schools. The report incorporates inputs from various expert individuals and organisations and a 1000-respondent survey to understand the issues prevalent within UK schools that lead to hair discrimination. Findings showed that 41% of children with Afro hair want to change their hair from curly to straight, and 1 in 6 children are having a bad or very bad experience at school connected to their Afro-textured hair. Anti-Afro hair policies in the UK appear to have risen by 66.7%, and WAD recommends that a review is conducted of all school policies in the UK to ensure that they do not breach equality guidelines when it comes to rules around hair in their uniform policies.

This action may prevent there being further cases like Ruby's, which can have a huge negative impact on a young person's life.

INTERVIEW WITH WORLD AFRO DAY CO-FOUNDER, MICHELLE DE LEON

ZKS: How and why did you start World Afro Day?

MDL: I was lying in my bed and I heard this singing from the bathroom. I think my daughter was about eight. And she was singing about how thankful she was for her Afro hair. I thought it was amazing, she was saying 'I'm a princess, I'm amazing' and I couldn't believe what I was hearing. I thought 'wow, I never felt that good about my hair'. The second thought that came to me was 'there's so many other children that don't feel that way'. In that moment, I felt connected to, beyond my own child, millions of other children around the world that don't feel good about their hair.

At the same time, I was seeing and hearing about all the pain and dissatisfaction of women around the world. So I had those two clear viewpoints; my daughter's celebration and the struggle around the world.

So, what about a day where we come together and share the positives and that becomes a marker for the future? It becomes a [day] where we say we're going to move forward, we're going to stop sharing the negative legacy of the past and we're going to create something that will empower, celebrate, uplift us and create momentum.

ZKS: What are your thoughts of the impact you have seen so far, since the inception of WAD. What was the impact of the year 2020 in particular?

MDL: The year 2020 had to matter more because of what we've been through; the pandemic, the deaths of George Floyd and Chadwick Boseman. These are major events that have happened to our community. The climate is such that everything to do with us matters more, every experience we're going through is painful and our voices are getting louder.

So, with our hair, it has been a cry for justice, [...] the treatment of our hair is now something that we are telling wider society is unacceptable. As a people, we have tolerated and accepted that our hair is not considered equal, we haven't fought for it as much as we needed to.

Now, I think we're ready to fight. We are seeing laws, such as the Crown Act in the US, being passed in the house of representatives because people decided that they were going to fight hair discrimination.

ZKS: Do you feel like part of the solution could be

more Black teachers or more Black people in education/policy making?

MDL: I don't think Black teachers can solve the problem because we don't know where they're at with their own hair journey. We cannot make the assumption that just because someone is Black that they are pro-natural hair. The school system is about educating people with the power, whether they're Black or white. Discriminating against our children is not acceptable. We can't guarantee that Black teachers would write different policies.

ZKS: With WAD, self-love and the recent natural hair movement, do you feel that we are seeing an impact and shift amongst the younger generation?

MDL: Social media still has a massive preference towards blonde, straight hair. I see a lot of young people with long straight hair. I call it the princess syndrome. As young people, our first exposure to hair is seeing a princess in a book. And I think there's a lot of little girls who never escaped the princess syndrome, and we carry that into our adult life. It's a seed that gets planted really early. And social media makes that syndrome worse.

But there is definitely progress because there is now knowledge, and skills are being shared. It's about loving your hair type and loving yourself—what springs from that will overflow into society.

As Black people, we're no longer changing our hair as a response to society—we're doing it in a response to self-love and self-acceptance.

ZKS: What challenges did you face when starting World Afro Day?

MDL: There was more ignorance when we first started; the goal was alway to change society and break the barriers that made us hate our hair. Black people have always known that we have this problem. So it was the wider society that needed to know, so that they could be a part of the change, and the normalisation of our hair.

There were conversations or situations where we were talking to people who didn't understand, but we had to be determined. People laughing out of ignorance was the most infuriating [because] they were laughing about our pain, which I found particularly gruelling.

Some people had genuinely never heard of [discrimination against Black hair] happening. I believed it was important to counteract this by getting professors and academics involved every year to ensure people understand that this is a real issue.

ZKS: When the report came out, how was it received?

MDL: There's a gulf between the media and the education system. The education system has not properly responded to the report yet, but we might have a conversation here and there about it.

If they'd read the report, then every headteacher or policymaker would at least be informed. The report has not quite found its place in terms of creating change, but it's a tool that can be used to take steps towards making that change. It received media coverage, but [its intended audience of] headteachers and policymakers have not received it yet. Ofsted and the unions did not respond, so we're going to keep talking about this until they respond.

ZKS: What is one achievement that you are really proud of?

MDL: The most important thing that WAD has done is the top 10 model competition. It's about giving young people the opportunity to talk about and celebrate their hair. [Seeing] little Black children celebrate their hair... made you feel good about yourself and them, that they were free enough to embrace who they were.

It's rare that we see ourselves loving ourselves... These children had a way to express their love and beauty. We never had something like that, so other kids could look at themselves and know they are wonderful the way that they are.

We chose ten models instead of one, so that young people have multiple role models that they can identify with. We need massive events like this to lift us up, and it has to be more than one individual that we are celebrating.

We need our global village to be lifting up our kids.

A few months later, I receive an email from Michelle:

'We felt that it was important to update you yon our breakthrough. Five major UK Teaching Unions are backing World Afro Day to end Afro hair discrimination in schools, including the ASCL, NAHT, Voice the Union, NEU and NASUWT. There will be ongoing collaboration with the unions and teacher resources will be provided by World Afro Day. We challenged them to end hair discrimination in 30 days and most of the unions responded to our call.'

4

DON'T TOUCH MY HAIR

MICROAGGRESSIONS

We've looked at the politics of Black women's hair, the challenges they face as a result, and the subsequent hair discrimination they experience. Going back to the 'Black British Women and their hair' survey, when participants were asked whether they had experienced hair discrimination, 43% of survey respondents said yes, with 35% stating that they were not sure and only 22% asserting that they did not.

When asked to share experiences and situations where participants may have faced hair discrimination, a large number of responses began with the phrase, 'I'm not sure if I have been discriminated against because of my hair, but…' followed by examples of microaggressions towards their hair.

The term 'microaggression' was coined by American psychiatrist Chester M. Pierce in the 1970s.[1] His precise definition was the 'subtle insults (verbal, nonverbal and/or visual) directed toward people of colour, often automatically or unconsciously.'[2] Today, the definiton has expanded to include subtle or indirect insults, actions and statements made against a marginalised group, subjecting them to often unintentional discrimination.

Microaggressions are not blatant forms of discrimination. They are covert in their nature, which means that people often question the validity or truth behind such claims. It also means that it can be difficult to identify when a microaggression has occurred, particularly in an environment where racism and discrimination are systemic. For many, discrimination is seen as clear, loud and direct such as a gay couple being asked to leave a venue because they are making people feel uncomfortable, or a Black person being called a racial slur whilst walking down the street. However, when it comes to discrimination and prejudice, the reality is it is far more nuanced than that. Discrimination often takes the form of snide remarks, backhanded comments and questionable actions.

Another characteristic of microaggressions is that they do not always occur with the intention to offend or hurt an individual. Instead, they often represent subconscious perceptions of a said person or group. An example of a microaggression that would fit this definition is when people tell Black women 'you have nice hair for a Black girl'. Such a comment is rooted in the same ideology that leads to people deeming Black hair as unprofessional or inferior, the same ideology that when left unchecked leads to hair discrimination, leads to horrible situations like Ruby's. Yet often, the people making a statement of this nature don't mean harm by it; indeed, they may think that they are offering a compliment to the individual. Such a comment can really only exist in a racially discriminative framework where Black hair represents something that is undesirable.

Of all the microaggressions Black women sporting natural hair (or any hairstyle for that matter) have faced, I would bet money on the most common one being hair-touching! This commonly frequented invasion of privacy is something that any Black girl or woman who wears their natural hair is familiar with. I, for one, have lost count of how many times it has happened to me. A 2020 study conducted by hair care brand Pantene discovered that 93% of Black people with Afro hair have experienced hair-related microaggressions. Fifty-three percent said that their natural hair had been judged as unattractive and unprofessional, and 46% of those surveyed had experienced uninvited hair touching.[3]

The 'Black British Women and their hair' survey was replete with anecdotes about everyday microaggressions that Black women face relating to their hair.

'I have had management "subtly" tell me how to wear my hair by complementing one hairstyle (eurasian weave) but criticising another style (canerows and braids).'

'I have been mistaken for another Black colleague because we both change our hairstyles often. I have also had people thinking how my hair is done makes me more "sassy" or gives me more of an "attitude".'

'I was even asked by a white female colleague (who apparently was a former hairdresser!) if I (and other Black women) wash my hair. She then proceeded to state the stereotype of "Black hair doesn't grow long." She had said they had one lesson on Black hair when she had trained, which is appalling and evidently not enough.'

Racial microaggressions such as the ones listed above are particularly harmful as they happen very often. Over time, the cumulative impact of such assaults has huge psychological effects.[4] These effects are often unseen by others, leading to those who experience them feeling as though they are second-class citizens. This can lead to a negative impact on self-esteem and an increase in self-doubt, particularly when trying to identify and report racist or harmful incidents.[5]

CULTURAL APPROPRIATION

'KYLIE JENNER ACCUSED OF CULTURAL APPROPRIATION FOR WEARING HAIR IN TWISTS'

'ADELE ACCUSED OF "CULTURAL APPROPRIATION" AFTER WEARING JAMAICAN BIKINI AND BANTU KNOTS IN HER HAIR'

'BRISTOL UNIVERSITY STUDENTS ACCUSED OF "BLACKING UP" AFTER WEARING CORNROW BRAIDS FOR FANCY DRESS PARTY'

The curious case of cultural appropriation has been at the centre of many debates in recent years. Every month, the online world seems to descend into chaos trying to get to the bottom of whether someone's behaviour is appropriating the culture of a minority group. From an ignorant tweet to an embarrassing photo, people's actions are increasingly being scrutinised on social media.

Cultural appropriation is a term used to describe the adoption and extraction of resources, creative forms, styles, or practices of people from another culture or identity. The framework for cultural appropriation to occur relies heavily on unequal power dynamics, namely a dominant culture taking from a minority or marginalised group or culture. Generally speaking, cultural appropriation works to remove the cultural context of the resource, practice or style in question with appropriators often praised for adopting or even creating the culture, whereas the group that it originates from are vilified or criticised for the same thing.

Cultural appropriation can often be conflated with the term 'cultural exchange', which is understood to be a mutual sharing of cultures and traditions across different groups. Cultural exchange is often viewed as a value to society, connecting and enriching communities equally. On the contrary, cultural appropriation is not.

How does appropriation relate to Black hair? Sadly, in more ways than I would hope for.

The Kardashian-Jenner family are usually at the centre of some form of cultural appropriation scandal being discussed on social media. An example of this occurred at the start of 2018, when Kim Kardashian shared a photo of herself wearing Fulani braids, a particular style of cornrows originating from the West African Fulani tribe.[6] Instead of calling them by their real name, Kim Kardashian instead opted to refer to the hair style as 'Bo Derek braids', crediting the Caucasian actress Bo Derek who wore these braids in the 1979 film *10*.[7]

Following Kim Kardashian's baptism of the hairstyle as 'Bo Derek braids', came the wave of magazines, videos and news stories all referring to the hairstyle just as she did. As expected, parts of the online Black community were not pleased and took to the internet to explain why Kardashian's dubbing of the braids incorrectly was harmful to the wider community of Black women.

Fulani braids have been worn by Black women for centuries, and whilst Black women are mocked, bullied, excluded from school or fired from their jobs because of such hairstyles, Kim Kardashian was praised for making this look a cool, new trend. Interestingly, the white actress who was the muse for Kardashian's look, Bo Derek, was similarly credited for creating a 'cross cultural wave' when she wore the hairstyle back in the '70s.[8]

In this scenario, Kardashian aided in completely erasing the role and history of Black women in this context by wrongly celebrating a white woman as the creator of a historic Black hairstyle.

Another issue with cultural appropriation is that appropriators can pick and choose when they want to dabble in the non-dominant culture without any repercussions. This is what is meant by the saying 'everyone wants to be Black but nobody wants to be Black',[9] or 'they want our rhythm but not our blues'. Both sayings grapple with the sentiment that non-Black people are often happy to engage, consume, enjoy Black culture, style, music and art yet in the same instance can harbour racist beliefs or make no effort to learn about the plight or history of the community.

If we apply this lens to the Kardashian-Fulani scandal, we can understand Kardashian as seemingly enjoying the Black hairstyle of Fulani braids, finding it aesthetically pleasing and fashionable, yet in the same instance, she did not read up on the origins of the style and correctly credit the marginalised community from which the style originated from.

Ultimately, celebrating and embracing different cultures is a good thing as long as it is not disadvantageous to the group that the culture originates from.

Some of you may be thinking, 'HOLD UP, wait a minute... When Black women straighten their hair, wear wigs or dye their hair blonde, are they appropriating white culture?' The answer is no. Historically speaking, these were all instances of cultural assimilation. As previously explored, for many years, Black women did not have a choice but to change their hair for economic security, social mobility and, quite frankly, survival. That is not to say that today, all Black women wear weaves or straighten their hair to assimilate into society, but historically speaking, this was certainly the case. Also, importantly, the actions of Black women in this instance is not detrimental or exploitative towards white people. With that context in mind, Black women altering, changing their hair in these ways is not a case of cultural appropriation.

BLACKFISHING

Blackfishing is a relatively recent phenomenon that gained popularity around 2018. Often referred to as modern-day blackface, blackfishing is a term coined by journalist Wanna Thompson. It is a spin on the word 'catfishing', which describes a person who deceives others online, usually by creating a fake persona or lying about aspects of their lives in an attempt to develop a relationship with an unassuming person.

Someone who participates in blackfishing tries to accentuate or imitate certain features so they appear to have Black heritage for social and often financial gain. Blackfishing is seen as problematic as it permits an individual to select the 'attractive' parts of being Black without facing the prejudice, racism and general plight of the Black community.

Many well-known white celebrities and influencers have increasingly been accused of Blackfishing and criticised for intentionally exploiting or taking advantage of the 'exotic' look of historically marginalised groups, sometimes to gain access to Black spaces.

In many cases of Blackfishing, modified hair plays a large role along with modified skin tone and facial features. In the cases where hair is employed, Caucasian hair is altered to appear 'Blacker', through use of braided styles, curls and more. A well known example of this is the case of Rachel Dolezal, perhaps one of the most infamous cases of Blackfishing in the modern age. To be quite honest, Rachel Dolezal's case is so complex and extreme, it may warrant a whole new term separate to blackfishing.

Rachel Dolezal is a former American college activist known for identifying as a Black woman when her heritage was, in fact, that of a white person. Dolezal was born as a blue-eyed, blonde, straight-haired white girl in Montana.[10] Part of the reason why Dolezal's case was perplexing was the lengths she went to, to pass as 'Black', which included tanning her skin and wearing a curly weave or braids.

Hair was a strong point of interest when it came to the Rachel Dolezal story. How did she get her hair to look so authentically Black? Who did it? So much so that when she finally did a CNN tell-all interview in 2015 and revealed that she wore a weave, social media exploded with conservation around the matter.[11]

So as you can see, the hair appropriation, blackfishing and microaggressions that Black women face are deeply complex. It is important for us to understand why these things happen and what can be done to stop them.

I will end this chapter on one of the anecdotes shared in the 'Black British Women and their hair' survey.

> 'I think Black women's hair is constantly appropriated, adopted, copied, latched onto like crazy and NEVER actually appreciated when it's on a Black woman's head other than by other Black women. Like, it's crazy to me that non-Black people say, "oh it's just a hairstyle"??? Okay, when Black people can exist without their hair being ridiculed, demeaned and discriminated against in all facets of society, only then will I think it's just a hairstyle...'

5

REPRESENTATION
SEEING IS BELIEVING

n the 'Black British Women and their hair' survey, 60% of participants selected mainstream media as a negative influence on their hair journey. Some anecdotes from the survey are below.

> 'Mainstream media has taught me that straight hair
> is the standard for beauty. Mainstream media lacks
> diversity, which shows me that the way my natural hair
> grows isn't what society sees as beautiful. It's progressing
> but has a LONG way to go.'

> 'Seeing Black women in the media with long, silky hair
> growing up, I didn't realise they were wearing wigs or
> chemically straightened their hair.'

As a young Black girl with Afro hair, the media's lack of representation of your hair type not only makes you feel unattractive or undesirable, but it also makes you feel completely erased.

Over the years, we have begun to see more Black people (and therefore more Black hair) in popular culture. I should admit, I am very cognisant when I do see a new Black face on television, in a magazine, on an advert and even more so if I see natural hair displayed. The feeling is an odd one. It is somewhere in between shock, joy and skepticism, and I am sure many other Black people can relate.

TV AND FILM

Before the early 1900s, there were no Black people in entertainment. The only time a Black character would appear on TV was in the form of white actors painting their faces black and acting like caricatures of Black people, a racist practice better known as blackface.

In 1946, Jamaican-born Pauline Henriques became the first Black woman to appear on British television. Born in Jamaica, Pauline Henriques came to Britain with her family in 1914 when she was five years old, and she displayed a love for acting from a very young age.[1] When she was 18, Henriques attended the London Academy of Music and Dramatic Art, where she enrolled in a drama course. It would be here that she would get to perfect her acting even further.

Henriques's race proved to be an obstacle when attempting to play roles at the academy, so she had to whiten her face when playing characters like Lady Macbeth.[2] Henriques's big break came about when she was cast in a BBC show called *All God's Chillun' Got Wings*, which first aired on 16th September 1946.[3] The show was based on an expressionist play by the same name about a dysfunctional interacial marriage where the white wife abuses her Black husband. The dominant theme of the play is racism, which for the BBC at the time would have been seen as a controversial move.

During this time, blackface was still popular, so even for someone like Pauline, it was difficult to secure acting roles due to competition from white actors who were 'blacking up'. Pauline, conscious of the obstacles faced by Black actors and actresses of her time, created the Negro Theatre Company to provide Black people with production opportunities.[4] Pauline Henriques spoke about how she had to 'whiten up' to secure acting roles—both in the way that she spoke and in her appearance. Even after her time in drama school, she would find that she was only given the role of Black maids with one line, 'Yessum. I'sa coming!' which she said she learned to say in 18 different ways.[5]

In America, Cicely Tyson became the first African-American woman to star in a TV drama *East Side/West Side* in 1963. She wore her natural hair out and cut short, a style now commonly called the TWA (teeny weeny afro). Tyson broke many norms—being a Black woman starring on TV for one, and also for wearing her natural hair. This went against the beauty norms of that period. During the heights of her career, Tyson sported a range of Black hairstyles, unapologetically displaying the versatility of Black hair. To date, many Black women, including actress Viola Davis, credit Tyson for helping them feel good about their Black skin and natural hair.

Pam Grier is said to be the first African-American actress to star in an action movie. Grier would play the iconic character of Foxy Brown in the 1974 film also called *Foxy Brown*. The famed scene of the movie sees Grier's character pull out a small gun hidden in her afro much to the surprise of her character's enemies. Foxy Brown as a character spearheaded the badass woman action hero and worked to challenge the gender stereotypes that dominated TV and film at that time. The character would go on to inspire a generation, leading to Beyoncé's character in *Austin Power* named Foxxy Cleopatra and rapper Foxy Brown naming herself after the character.

In 1968, Barbara Blake-Hannah became the first Black female news reporter on British TV.[6] Like Henriques, Blake-Hannah was Jamaican-born and from a wealthy background. Her arrival at Thames Television sparked a lot of attention for good and bad reasons, with many people not comfortable with seeing a Black reporter on TV. Blake-Hannah was oblivious to the storm her arrival in the TV world was causing, partly because she was busy enjoying her job and colleagues.

Eventually, however, Blake-Hannah began to experience racism, which ended up impacting her career. As part of a news feature, she was asked to swim in a pool alongside a white reporter. Blake-Hannah was a very strong swimmer but had straightened her hair for filming that would take place later that day. She did the breaststroke, taking extra care to keep her hair out of the water so it would stay straight. The fact that she swam like this was used in the feature as proof that Black people could not swim as well as white people.[7]

It was a particularly tricky time for race relations and only nine months after securing her job as a reporter, Thames Television decided to let Blake-Hannah go because they were receiving too many complaints from viewers who did not approve of seeing a Black woman on their screens. It would be 13 years later that we would see more Black female representation, with Moira Stewart hitting TV screens as a BBC news reporter, regularly sporting her hair in an afro or a straight pixie cut.

All of this was before my time, and I cannot imagine how challenging it must have been for young Black girls to grow up with almost no representation back then. I grew up in '90s Britain, and whilst the representation of Black women in the media left a lot to be desired, I do feel lucky to have experienced the few Black women that did grace my TV screen. Seeing Angelica Bell on BBC's *Blue Peter* and June Sarpong on Channel 4's *T4* meant the world to me. During this time, it was still rare to see a Black woman on TV with her natural hair out. Gradually, this has changed, and we are seeing more hair diversity on screen. Black women like Charlene White presenting the ITV News with a twist out and Judi Love and Clara Amfo presenting TV shows with their natural hair loose or in braids, all add to promoting and representing Black women and Black hair in its versatility.

Seeing Black people in the media is only one aspect of representation. Being presented with stories that relate to our experiences as Black people is another. In the 21st century, the conversations around Black hair have become notably louder.

Chris Rock's 2009 documentary *Good Hair* is one of the most well-known documentaries that explores Black hair in America. Inspired to make the film after his daughter told him that she was upset that she didn't have 'good hair', the documentary takes Chris Rock on a journey through various US states and to India, interviewing experts and prominent African-Americans to better understand Black hair and the complexities that come with it.

Although the documentary covered important topics such as the chemicals found in hair relaxers, the hair industry and the skill of hairstyling in an informative and often comedic way, in my opinion, it failed to acknowledge certain aspects of Black hair care today, and the pressures Black women face to conform to societal norms.

The documentary talks about how Black women 'want to be white' and spend ridiculous amounts of money on wigs and weaves without exploring the nuances as to why Black women may feel the need to do this. The documentary seems to almost blame Black women for their decision to relax their hair or wear extensions.

The history of Black hair is also now being told through various mediums. In March 2020, Netflix released a four-part series called *Self Made*, telling the story of Madame CJ Walker's life.

Later that year in October, Channel 4 aired the documentary *Hair Power: Me and My Afro* by Emma Dabiri, author of *Don't Touch My Hair*. The show explored the hair stories and journeys of Black people in modern Britain. The 2018 romcom, *Nappily Ever After*, follows the journey of Violet as she breaks up with her boyfriend and realises that she was never truly herself around him. As part of this, he never saw her natural hair because she always straightened it. There is a particularly dramatic scene where she shaved her head off, symbolising the start of her new journey to self-love and turning her back on the societal pressure that forced her to straighten her hair. The film has some emotional moments but is generally quite light-hearted.

The 2020 film *Bad Hair* is a comedy-horror where a woman gets a weave to succeed in the television industry. However, she realises that her weave 'has a mind of its own', and it is possessed! The film received mixed reviews.

THIS is what I want to see more of. Black hair as the hero, Black hair as the villain, Black hair as the love interest. Top-quality educational pieces about Black hair and silly, funny films about Black hair. I want it all.

FASHION INDUSTRY

The prevailing norms of the fashion industry often set the standard for how beauty is defined. More often than not, this ideal is exclusionary, non-diverse and unachievable. When we assess the fashion industry's relationship to Black women and their hair, we uncover that the industry is often fertile ground for texturism, natural hair discrimination, colourism and racism.

Despite the large number of professionals who work in fashion, the lack of Black hairstylists in the industry combined with the lack of education on natural Black hair means that Black models are often subject to traumatic experiences including microaggressions and hair discrimination. Stacey Ciercon, a hair expert, once stated that as a result of this environment, models feel like they cannot voice their opinions due to concerns about job security.[8]

Black models have spoken out about the fashion industry's problematic relationship with Black hair. In 2015, model Jordan Dunn revealed that hairstylists in the industry have damaged her hair because they did not know how to handle Afro hair.[9] She would go on to reveal that she had lost all hair around her hairline and had to wear wigs as a result of the damage.[10]

Model Leomie Anderson has also been vocal about how Black women and their hair are treated in the modelling industry. Anderson reported noticing her white counterparts get their hair and make-up done for two hours, whereas the stylists would only spend 10 minutes on her because no-one had the appropriate beauty products. She would go on to call this experience 'incredibly demorisaling.'[11]

Anderson explained that experiences like Fashion Week can be traumatic for Black models, admitting that Black models can have three or four shows per day, having their hair styled and re-styled by a person who does not care about their hair's needs.[12] Anderson states that she has seen cases of Black models who start Fashion Week with healthy hair, only to have it completely damaged by the end of it, as it happened to her where she lost two inches of hair in one month due to how her hair was treated backstage.[13]

Similarly, model Olivia Anakwe took to Instagram in 2019 during Paris Fashion Week, calling out stylists who don't know how to handle Black hair, making the point that, 'Black hair-stylists are required to know how to do everyone's hair, why does the same not apply to others?'[14] Anakwe would go on to detail how hairstylists would turn their backs on her as she approached them, and one lady pulled on her edges harshly in an attempt to cornrow her hair.[15] Her post read, 'I was ignored, I was forgotten and I felt that.'[16]

Anakwe, Dunn and Anderson are not the first models to experience such a hostile environment in the fashion industry when it comes to natural Black hair, and they likely will not be the last. Even fashion icon Naomi Campbell has spoken about having to provide her own hair and make-up products at photoshoots when she first began modelling.[17] The fashion industry's intolerant attitude towards Black hair has long been felt by Black models and industry observers, but until the necessary changes take place such as hiring more Black hairstylists and educating all hairstylists on how to care for Black hair, this will remain a pervasive issue.

Alek Wek is a South-Sudanese-born model who moved to London when she was 14. A dark-skinned Black woman with short hair, the high fashion world was drawn to her unique look and South-Sudanese features.[18] In 1998, Wek modelled in a Betsey Johnson runway show, where all models were sporting straight blonde wigs. When Wek got to the end of the catwalk, she ripped the wig off her head and threw it into the audience. This move would go on to make a loud statement in the fashion industry and beyond. For many, Wek, a Black woman, throwing off a blonde wig was symbolic of the rejection of the white beauty standards that pervades the fashion industry. Wek later reflected on this moment in an interview saying, 'that wig was not just about me taking it off to make a scene. It was a time that I was just starting in fashion... And the one thing that I told my agents was if you are going to represent me, I'm not going to be a gimmick and be in for a couple of seasons. You're going to take it all or leave it.'[19] To Wek, it wasn't enough to just be a Black model. She was not going to be a token and her success was not going to be defined by how closely she could align herself to Eurocentric beauty standards.

In 2016, a report published by *The Fashion Spot* revealed that 78.2% of all the models featured in spring 2016's fashion adverts were white, and only 8.3% of models were Black.[20] Statistics like these are sadly not shocking. They highlight that until Black representation within the fashion industry increases, both on the runway and behind the scenes, Black people and their hair in all its versatility will not be fully accepted and championed.

Now let's go back to the '60s, back to the Black Power Movement in the US. As we discussed in Chapter 3, with this movement came an aesthetic change in the form of Black people increasingly wearing their natural hair. Whilst for Black people of that time this change was a political statement in favour of Black freedom and pride, for non-Black communities, the infamous image of The Black Panther Party would later become just a fashionable look. The Black Panthers, aesthetically speaking, were known for their all-militant image with black clothing, black berets, black gloves, black leather jackets and natural hair, so much so that this image has become synonymous with the Black Power Movement as a whole. Years after the group's prominence, this image would become even more popular with the fashion industry, bringing The Black

Panther Party style onto the catwalk. Beyoncé's 2016 Super Bowl performance was an ode to the Black Panthers, with her and her dancers donning afros and black berets.

The popularisation of the image of Black people with their natural hair has resulted in Afro hair being employed as a prop and a costume by those outside of the Black community. In the fashion industry, this has happened in the form of white models donning Afro-looking hair. In August 2015, magazine *Allure* published a feature piece on 'how to get an afro'. The model who was casted for the piece was a white model who appeared to have Afro-textured hair. The article called the style a 'loose afro' and detailed how people, including those with straight hair, could attain the afro look.[21] The photo of the white model would cause a Twitter storm, with readers noting that the article did not mention Black women or the history and context surrounding the afro.

In 2017, the UK magazine *Blackhair* released its December/January issue, which had a cover featuring white and Malaysian model Emily Bador with her hair styled like an afro.[22] The photo itself appeared edited in a way that meant it was not clear that the model was not Black, nevertheless, when the model's race was revealed, the magazine and the model came under fire. The model herself released a statement apologising, directing her statement at Black women, explaining that the shoot occurred when she was a teenager and had no understanding of the experience of women of colour and cultural appropriation.[23]

In 2018, *Vogue* came under criticism for printing a photo of model Kendall Jenner in what people saw as an afro-style hairstyle.[24] Jenner was in two photos with the afro-style hair, one photo alongside Black model Imaan Hammam, whose hair was straight. *Vogue* responded by apologising for any offence caused, stating that the look was meant to evoke the feel of the early 20th century.[25]

The list really does go on and it extends onto the catwalk, where fashion designers select white models to walk the runway wearing Afro-textured wigs or altering their hair to appear as though it has an Afro texture. Usually, after the backlash, designers and models apologise for the offence caused, yet it continues to happen.[26] Afros are not the only Black hairstyles that are subject to fall appropriation by the fashion industry—dreadlocks, braids and cornrows all suffer similar fates.

MUSIC

In 1939, Evelyn Dove would become the first Black female singer to be on BBC radio.[27]

Evelyn Dove was born in 1902 to an affluent family in London. Her father was a barrister from Sierra Leone and her mother was English. Evelyn was privately educated and became a successful cabaret performer, eventually touring Europe and gaining popularity in America.[28]

A couple of decades later in the '50s, Winifred Atwell, a concert pianist from Trinidad and Tobago, would study at the Royal Academy of Music and become the first Black person to sell a million records in Britain and have a number one hit in the UK.[29]

Interestingly, when we assess Black women such as Atwell, Dove, Henriques and Blake-Hannah who were the 'first' to achieve an accolade or position of success and power in the 1900s, we find that they were often from relatively privileged backgrounds. Herein lies the intersection and interaction that race and class present when it comes to the outcome of an individual's life. This appears to be more prevalent in the arts and media sector, perhaps because public perception and sentiment plays a huge role in the success of in this space.

Nowadays, the barrier to entry into numerous industries has lowered, perhaps because there is more pressure on companies to diversify their workforce. Now, we are seeing people of all racial and socioeconomic backgrounds pursuing careers and thriving, with companies beginning to encourage and embrace this diversity.

The music industry has a deep history of colourism, overlooking dark-skinned Black women in favour of lighter-skinned women. Some of the most popular and successful Black women artists (see: Beyoncé, Rihanna, Nicki Minaj and similarly in the UK, Stefflon Don and Jorja Smith) are light skinned, with looser hair textures and often wear wigs, weaves and extensions. This is not to say that there are not successful and popular dark-skinned Black women artists, because there are. However, the dominant and mainstream face of Black women artistry is the archetypal light-skinned woman. This image and its relative proximity to whiteness provides lighter-skinned musicians an advantage over darker-skinned artists as their aesthetic holds social value within mainstream culture. In turn, it provides them with greater access to the music industry and success. Take Beyoncé, for example, who is one of the most well known musicians of our time (and rightfully so!). Beyoncé is known for her talent, work ethic, beautiful voice, brilliant choreography and her extensive musical catalogue. She is also known for her looks, which to many are seen as the pinnacle of mainstream Black beauty. Beyoncé is a full figured, light-skinned woman with Eurocentric phenotypes who regularly sports long, blonde wigs. When asked if Beyoncé's career would have been more challenging had she been darker-skinned, Beyoncé's father and ex-manager, Mathew Knowles, admitted that it would have affected her success.[30] Before you hardcore Beyoncé fans come for my neck,

I would like to say on record that I believe that she is one of the greatest performers of all time. However, to not acknowledge the role that her appearance and its proximity to whiteness has played in her career would be dishonest.

When we look at important Black British musicians, specifically, in relation to Black hair, we must start with Mel B. Mel B was a member of the Spice Girls, one of the most successful girl groups of all time. Nicknamed 'Scary Spice', she was known for her big curly afro and her colourful outfits. Mel B was the first celebrity whom I came across in my childhood that I felt I could relate to because, just like me, her hair spiralled out in all directions. Combined with her bold personality and unapologetic confidence, Scary Spice made me feel like my hair texture was to be celebrated and not hidden.

Mel B was the only Black girl in an otherwise all-white pop group. Her nickname Scary Spice was established by a white male journalist, who gave nicknames to each of the members when the band first started.[31] The nickname begs the question, what exactly is scary about Mel B? Her skin? Her natural hair? Her confidence? Or maybe all three? One cannot ignore the racial connotations behind dubbing a confident unapologetic Black woman with natural hair as scary. Now, it may be the case that the journalist who created the nickname did not do so to be intentionally demeaning or offensive. Mel B herself is on record taking no offence to the nickname and publicly embracing it. Nevertheless, labelling a Black girl with natural hair and a strong personality as 'scary' does in fact build on pre-existing stereotypes of Black women and natural Black hair.

In 2020, following the Black Lives Matter protests sparked by the death of George Floyd, many Black celebrities began to speak out about the racism they had faced in their industries.

Mel B shared that when the Spice Girls were about to film the music video for their debut single, 'Wannabe', she was told that her hair needed to be straightened.[32] She refused to let this happen, stating, 'my hair was my identity and yes it was different to all the other girls, but that was what the Spice Girls were about—celebrating our differences.'[33]

Alexandra Burke, the 2008 winner of the TV talent show *X-Factor*, also spoke out in 2020 about the racism she experienced in the music industry.[34] She was advised that if she wanted to be successful, she would have to tone down her Blackness. 'I got told when I first won the X-Factor, "because you're Black, you're going to have to work 10 times harder than a white artist because of the colour of your skin. You can't have braids, you can't have an afro [...]. You have to have hair that appeals to white people so they understand you better."'[35]

To mark World Afro Day 2018 the BBC did a feature on singer Jamelia, where she was interviewed by her daughter Tiani about her hair.[36] When asked why her hair was straight throughout her music career, Jamelia explained that 'at the time, that was how Black singers had their hair and I wanted to be like everyone else.'[37] She talks about her idols, Mary J Blige, Monica, Aaliyah and Beyoncé all having straight weaves and feeling like that's what she needed to be successful.

Jamelia, inspired by her daughters and wanting to set an example, eventually cut off her hair and grew it back, keeping it all natural. Tiani explained that it was really exciting to see her mum with Afro hair because, 'we have the same hair and that means my hair is nice too.'[38]

Rochelle Humes, member of the British girl group The Saturdays, decided to embrace her curls after a conversation with her daughter, who came home from school upset that she couldn't be a princess because 'princesses only have straight hair'.[39] Humes realised that her daughter had never seen her hair in its natural curly state because she always blow-dried it. She cut off her damaged hair and grew her curls back, also publishing a children's book about curly hair to inspire and empower other young kids.[40]

This is the future of representation I hope for, calling out people, organisations and industries that are discriminatory towards Black women and Black hair, and taking action to make a real change and inspire future generations.

INTERVIEW FOUNDER OF PROJECT EMBRACE, LEKIA LEE

Due to the lack of representation of Black Afro-textured hair across the media, many groups and individuals have begun doing their bit to change the skewed playing field and give Black hair the representation that it deserves. One of these individuals is a woman by the name of Lekia Lee. Lekia Lee is the founder of Project Embrace, which is an initiative that creates positive visual media representation of Afro-textured hair and challenges the misrepresentation of Black women and their natural hair in the media, workplace and society at large, through billboard campaigns. I was lucky enough to speak to Lekia Lee about her own hair journey and what moved her to create Project Embrace.

ZKS: How would you describe your journey with your hair?

LL: My hair journey, should I say, came towards the end of a journey of acceptance. I was going through a period where I wanted to change the way I felt about myself because I didn't feel beautiful. I think, for a woman, that affects so many other aspects of your life, what you choose to do, who you choose to be and how you allow people to treat you. I remember being teased for being Black in school and I've always had to prove myself throughout my life and career. I just had to do something to change the way I was feeling and I began to work to regain my confidence. And it occurred to me that if I was on this journey of loving myself and seeing my worth, then why did I keep relaxing my hair? It didn't sit well with me. So I shaved everything. I wanted to tell the world that was telling me that I wasn't good enough, that I was good enough.

ZKS: What inspired you to start Project Embrace?

LL: I had been on this self-love journey for five years when I had my daughter, and I didn't want her to ever feel like how I felt. I could see the way that the media portrays women and Black women especially. The narrative out there wasn't going to empower her and validate her as a person. I didn't want her to ever feel like she had to conform to someone else's standard of beauty.

I was quite militant about the images and information that she received at home and she had only just started nursery. She was not a shy child, and I noticed that at just three-years-old she would only compliment women with either permed hair or straight weaves and wigs. But what made it so surprising was that at home, she didn't see any of those images. It made me realise how strong external influences are. I thought to myself, why don't I put messages out there on the streets, to show everyone that Black women with natural hair are beautiful as well.

That was my motivation to start Project Embrace. I want to inspire my daughter and, by extension, young Black girls like her. I wanted to challenge the idea of what it means to be beautiful and acceptable, and I wanted society to see Black women differently.

ZKS: What challenges did you face when starting up the billboard campaign?

LL: People would tell me that I'm creating a solution to a problem that doesn't exist and that women can wear their hair in whatever way they want to. I'm not saying you can't wear your hair in a particular way, I'm saying we should be able to do so without fear or concern about how others will view or treat us as a result.

If the majority of Black women feel they can't wear their natural hair or don't even see the beauty in their natural hair, then we need to fix this.

People always ask me 'why did you not just do a social media campaign which would have been much cheaper?' Social media uses algorithms. I didn't want the campaign to be shown only to people who might want to see it. I wanted everybody to see it whether they liked to or not. With a billboard, you HAVE to see it, you don't have a choice.

ZKS: What has the impact been?

LL: Young girls reaching out saying: 'I'm so happy that you're addressing this problem because it makes me feel like I'm of value.' Mothers contacting me to say that the campaign has boosted their daughters' confidence.

I've been quite overwhelmed by the impact. When the first campaign went out in 2017, the BBC picked it up, and it was on the six o'clock news. After that happened, it went much further than I anticipated and had even hoped for, and I even had the Washington Post call me from the States. I think this has opened up people's eyes to the unconscious bias they have towards Black women and how Black women look. This has helped that conversation to be opened up and people have the courage to speak about this.

ZKS: What is your goal with the Afrovisibility campaign?

LL: It's a big goal. I hope that we can use the Afrovisibility campaign to help heal the world of racism. And I think we're getting there, one step at a time. There are so many more voices and campaigns now shedding light on this issue. With the CROWN act, people are passing laws about this. The more voices we have, the louder we are and the greater impact we will make.

6

MONEY, BUSINESS AND THE BLACK HAIR INDUSTRY

Between 2016 and 2018, the Black hair industry in the UK was reported to be worth an estimated £88 million,[1] and in the US, the Black hair care industry was set to make $2.51 billion.[2] Here in the UK, Black British women spend between three and six times as much on their hair as white women (depending on what studies you are reading).[3][4] As part of the 'Black British Women and their hair' survey I conducted, I asked respondents to estimate how much they spend on their hair each year. Many responses mentioned that they've never really thought about this and can't comprehend it, knowing that they will be shocked at the reality of how much of their money goes towards their hair. Based on the estimates I did receive, it's extremely common for Black women to spend hundreds, if not thousands, of pounds on their hair each year.

One afternoon when I was hanging out with friends, I asked them what questions they have about the hair industry as Black women. Their questions ranged from:

> "Why can't I find products that work for my hair in high street shops?"

"Why are Black hair products more expensive than
mainstream brands?"

"Why does it feel like the Black hair industry is run by
non-Black people that don't understand our hair?"

For what is a booming industry with a lot of opportunity,
Black consumers often feel undervalued, with their needs not
being fully met. So, how did this happen and what is needed
to change this?

There is not a huge amount of research that exists today on
Black British consumers or businesses. UK research that is
available tends to look only at the BAME (Black, Asian and
minority ethnic) population. The acronym BAME provides a
rather broad and generalised category of non-white indenti-
ties. This is often more counterproductive than useful, as it
fails to acknowledge the nuances relating to different identities. When it comes to Black hair consumerism in particular,
this category is not very helpful as Black hair consumerism
is not an experience that is shared by other racial or ethnic
groups. It is thus essential that in our attempts to understand
the true experience of groups in the UK and beyond that we
do not simply push non-white identities together but, instead,
acknowledge the diversity and differences amongst the many
identities that exist.

A statistic I came across many times in my research for
this book was that the spending power of Black consumers in
the UK is approximately £300 billion.[5] This statistic comes
from a report called 'Multicultural Britain 2012' published by
the Institute of Practitioners in Advertising (IPA). However,
when you dig a bit deeper into this research, we find that this
number is actually the estimate for the purchasing power of

the BME population (Black and minority ethnic). Herein lies a real life example of how terms such as BAME or BME conflate the differences of non-white groups, preventing us from gaining accurate insight into the plethora of groups this term represents.

So, what are the facts? Well, we know that Black people have huge purchasing power and we also know that a lot of Black people's money is spent outside of the Black community. So, why do so many Black consumers still feel like they are an afterthought?

SHMONEY, POWER AND BUSINESS

As we explored in Chapter 2, Black entrepreneurs pioneered the Black hair care industry, with the likes of George E. Johnson and Dyke & Dryden creating products that made Black people feel acknowledged and seen. After seeing how profitable the Black hair industry was becoming, large white-owned manufacturers decided they wanted a piece of the pie, buying out Black-owned hair care brands as well as signing endorsement deals with well known Black celebrities to advertise their products.[6] This move would go on to change the once majority Black-owned Black hair care industry into an industry that would now be led by white-owned corporations.

In the late '60s, straightening products began to decline in sales, due to the rise of the Black Power Movement and the wider Black population in the West choosing to wear their natural hair instead of straightening and relaxing their hair.[7] With this change in consumer demand, existing Black businesses that focused on hair straightening products found themselves in a predicament. Many hairstylists and companies went out of business as a result, but Johnson Products expanded their product range to cater for natural hair too, introducing Afro Sheen,[8] managing to stay relevant in a changing market. In the UK, Dyke & Dryden Ltd also took the same approach, expanding their product range to include the 'afro comb'.

While this shift in the Black hair market continued, Joan and George E. Johnson stood their ground and Johnson Products managed to maintain their market share for a number of years. However, George E. Johnson eventually had to relinquish ownership of Johnson Products as part of his divorce settlement, and Joan sold the company to Ivax Corporation, which was, you guessed it, white-owned! It was later sold again to Carson Products in 1998, and then to Proctor & Gamble in 2003. In March 2009, Johnson Products was bought by RCJP Acquisition Inc,[9] a partnership between private equity firms Rustic Canyon/Fontis Partners LP, St. Cloud Capital and African-Americans Eric Brown and Renee Cottrell-Brown. This deal meant that Brown and Cottrell-Brown, who are husband and wife, became the new owners of Johnson Products, making it Black-owned again.[10]

Meanwhile, a similar story was unravelling for Dyke and Dryden Ltd. Dyke, Dryden and Wade had made a name for themselves and were dominating the Black hair care industry in the UK with their 'for us, by us' mindset. When the team decided that they wanted to sell the business, they hoped that young Black people in the community would take it over but, unfortunately, they could not find anyone to sell their business to. In 1987, Dyke & Dryden Ltd was acquired by American company Soft Sheen, one of the biggest Black hair brands in history, which had been created by African-Americans Edward and Bettiann Gardner. Soft Sheen was bought by L'Oréal in 1998.

White-owned conglomerates and companies have been accused of 'deception' when it comes to marketing their

Black hair care brands and products. This 'deception' lies in the fact that many feel that the marketing methods of these companies are created to intentionally imply they are Black-owned. In America, these concerns would lead to the creation of the American Health and Beauty Aids Institute (AHBAI) in 1981.[11] The Institute was created to represent, 'the thriving ethnic health and beauty care industry', with the institute making the point that the Black hair industry is one of the few industries in America that was created and founded by African-Americans.[12] The AHBAI would go on to create the globally recognised 'Proud Lady' symbol, a silhouette of a Black woman's head and hair which notifies consumers that a hair and beauty company is Black-owned.[13]

In 1992, there were numerous legal disputes within the hair industry in America,[14] including Shark Products Co. of Brooklyn, which is a white-owned conglomerate who created the Black hair product called 'African Pride'.[15] In the summer of 1992, the company would go on to sue not one, but two Black-owned companies, 'African Natural' and 'Mother Africa', alleging that the two companies had wrongfully copied their portrayal of the word 'African' and the 'African Pride' packaging.[16]

One case would be settled out of court in 1993, with the other being dropped altogether that same year. The cases marked a watershed moment for Black-owned companies, with many in the Black community seeing the lawsuits as a direct attack on Black ownership and Black businesses' right to use words like 'African' freely.

Similarly in Britain, the Black hair care industry was becoming less Black-owned. In a 2015 interview, Tony Wade of Dyke and Dryden Ltd reflected on the rise in Asian businesses entering the Black hair industry:

"The Asians saw something that was good. In fact, I used to supply them, they were coming to me and buying the largest quantities. You see, what we mustn't forget is that business is market-driven. If you are smart enough to provide what people want, they will go and get it from wherever they want. Our people have the same opportunities that Asian people have, but they didn't take the opportunities."[17]

Asian communities would have a reasonable presence in the Black hair care industry, producing many of the hair products that would be sold. Over time, the South Asian community in the UK would transition into selling the products, and today, it is rare for me to walk into a Black hair shop in London that is not South Asian-owned. There is not a huge amount of research around exactly how this transition happened, but I suspect it is a similar story to what happened in the US with the Korean community. Korean immigration into the US started in the '60s, and by using their connections in Asia, Koreans began to import hair products into America.[18] Over time, more and more Korean businesses entered the market to take advantage of this commercial opportunity.

The steady decline of the British empire would begin in 1945, with the independence of nations such as India in 1947, South Asian migration into the UK would rapidly increase during the 1950s and '60s, with migrants from nations such as Sri Lanka, India and Pakistan and modern-day Bangladesh entering the UK to start new lives. Perhaps, after the selling of Dyke & Dryden Ltd to Soft Sheen, this marked the beginning of non-Black businesses entering the UK Black hair care market. Similar to Koreans in the US, South Asians in the UK may have accessed manufacturers in their home countries to

CHAPTER 8: WHO DID YOUR HAIR?: THE WORLD OF HAIRSTYLING

AFRO

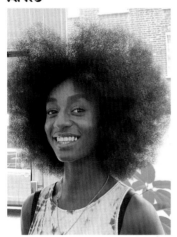

Zainab Kwaw-Swanzy

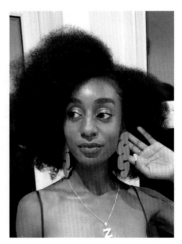

Zainab Kwaw-Swanzy taken by Kaiya John

WASH-AND-GO

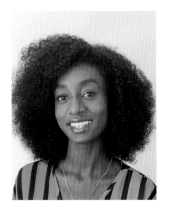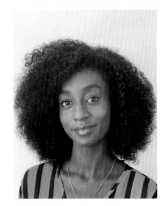

Zainab Kwaw-Swanzy taken by Zahra Swanzy

BLOWOUT

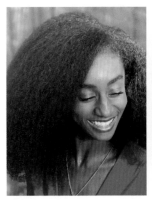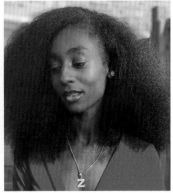

Zainab Kwaw-Swanzy taken by Zahra Swanzy

SILK PRESS

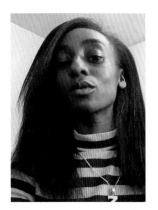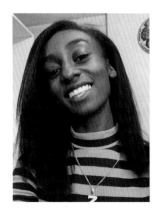

Zainab Kwaw-Swanzy

RELAXED

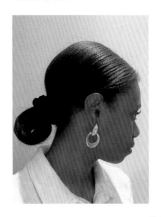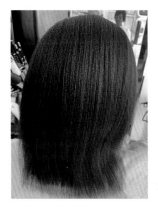

Eni Shobo

TWISTS

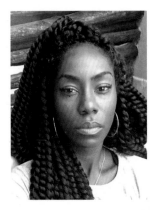 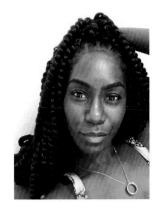

Zahra Swanzy

BANTU KNOTS

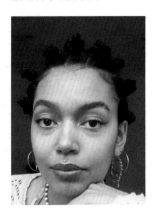 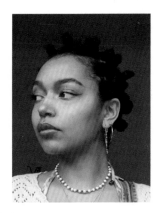

Sarah Hawke

BRAIDS/PLAITS

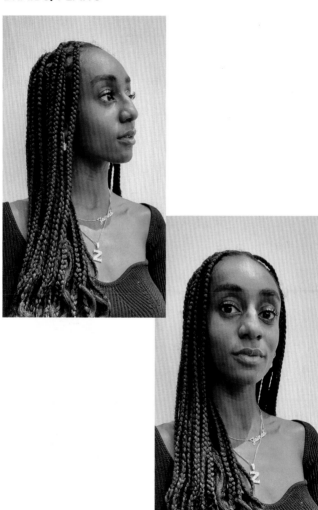

Zainab Kwaw-Swanzy taken by Daniel Carter

CANEROWS/CORNROWS

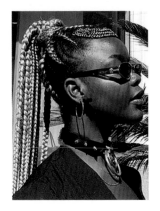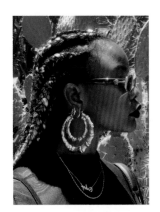

Liza Bakeyi

LOCKS

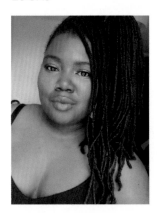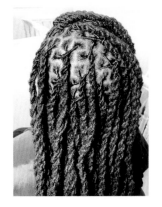

Sarauniya Shehu

WIGS/WEAVES

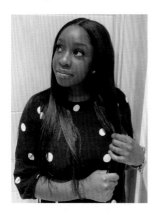 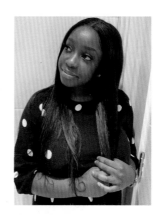

Julie Ssali by Zainab Kwaw-Swanzy

SHAVED

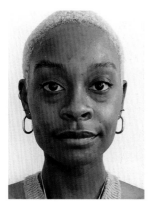 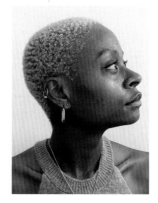

Yas Philgence

LAYING YOUR EDGES

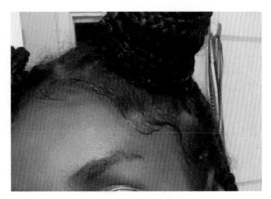

Zainab Kwaw-Swanzy

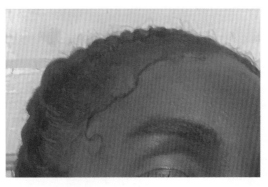

Zainab Kwaw-Swanzy

import and ultimately distribute Black hair products.

In the UK, if you need to buy anything relating to Black hair and beauty, 9 times out of 10, you will be recommended to check out Pak's. Established over 30 years ago, Pak's (full name Pak's Cosmetic Centre) is, 'Europe's leading supplier of multicultural hair & beauty products.' It is arguably the most popular and prominent chain of Black hair shops in London. Why has Pak's, an Asian-owned shop, become so successful and why haven't Black retailers managed to achieve that same scale?

If we take a step back, we will observe that most of the supply chain is Asian-owned. Many Black hair products are produced by Asian manufacturers, who are then responsible for the import and distribution of the products. It is then easy for them to also become retailers, since they are already connected to every other part of the supply chain. It's a fully connected network, allowing them to pool money together, increase their purchasing power and open more high street shops.

For someone wanting to open a Black hair shop, Dominique Lescott, founder of Hairpopp, an online marketplace for Black-owned hair brands in the UK, believes that there are two challenges they will face. When I interviewed her, she stated that, '[Black-owned businesses] don't have access to the relevant networks to buy stock, and the stock that they do manage to buy won't be sold to them at the price that it is sold to other ethnicities.'

Dominique explained that South Asian retailers will buy huge quantities together for a cheaper price, whereas the equivalent community doesn't exist for Black people, and so they are subject to higher prices from the wholesaler. What this means is that the Black retailer has to price their stock at an even higher price in order to make a profit. Black customers may enter an independent Black-owned hair shop and observe higher prices than in a superstore like Pak's, and therefore they may take their business to the place where prices are lower.

Dominique believes that the solution could be for Black retailers to imitate what the Asian ones have been doing for years. 'Black people need to be able to buy in bulk. The more you team up and buy collectively, the more it brings down your wholesale price. I haven't really seen this being done within the Black British hair care industry at all. When we begin to do that, we may have a lot more power within the industry and access to reduced prices.'

Sandra Brown-Pinnock founded xSandy's Hair and Beauty in 2015, making Sandy the only Black woman in (an incredibly diverse) Lewishman in South East London to run a hair shop. Prior to this, Sandy opened a hair salon in 2006 and created her own brand of hair extensions. In an interview with *gal-dem* magazine in 2018, Sandra spoke about her experience of going into a high street shop and the shopkeeper not being able to provide her with any appropriate product recom-mendations. She observed that most of the retail outlets in South East London were not owned by someone of African or Caribbean descent and wanted to make a change. For Sandra, it was not just about selling products. It was about equipping Black women with the right information and advice for their hair.

The Black hair product market in the US and UK has been dominated by a small number of brands, Dark and Lovely, Cantu, Eco Style, Creme of Nature to name a few. Two things that these brands have in common is that they exclusively specialise in products for Afro- or curly-textured hair types and they are not Black-owned. Despite these brands being extremely popular amongst Black women, there are concerns that the ingredients used in these products can be detrimental to Afro hair.

Between 2011 and 2018, the number of Black business owners in the UK increased by 98.6%, more than any other demographic.[19] Whilst we are now seeing an increase in Black-owned hair care brands, these companies face a number of challenges when entering the industry.

Many Black-owned hair brands have similar beginnings. The founder experimented with their own products, realised the benefits, shared them with friends and family and ultimately decided to make it a business. As these businesses are starting up, issues regarding the supply chain arise. There is the challenge of not being able to buy large quantities of raw ingredients, such that they're offered at a reduced price. Without these wholesale prices, small, independent businesses can't offer competitive prices to their customers.

In the case of newer brands that are focused on creating products that are good for Black hair, a lot of the raw materials used, such as shea butter and coconut oil, originate from African countries. In that sense, the whole process ultimately starts and ends with Black people—our countries produce the underlying ingredients and we are the consumers. However, with high barriers to entry and large conglomerates doing their best to dominate these supply chains, accessing this market can prove difficult for Black businesses. Despite this, Dominique Lescott of Hairpopp believes that this is an incredibly lucrative area, with Black people best equipped to exist in this space.

"There is a lot of money to be made throughout the supply chain. It's very important that we build our own networks so that we can then expand and keep that Black pound within our community."

Today, we are seeing more Black retailers and Black hair brands thriving. In London alone, we have seen Black-owned hair shops like Hair Glo in South East London, Hairitage in North West London, Golden Touch in East London and Mr Klass in North London amongst others. Across the UK, we have seen the success of Black-owned hair brands such as Afrocenchix, Big Hair, Afro Hair & Skin Co, Charlotte Mensah, Boucleme and others.

It is difficult to provide a sole reason as to why there appears to be a Black-owned boom in the hair industry, but it is likely to be a combination of varying factors. Social movements such as Black Lives Matter, combined with the general increase in societal consciousness around health, beauty and business have all played a role in Black consumers actively searching for independent hair brands and products that align with their values. People are now more likely to explore alternative companies with the intention to support local or minority communities. Within the UK specifically, Black British culture has risen in popularity and consequently financial viability, which has also contributed to the increase in appetite for Black-owned products.

The digital space has also provided an invaluable medium for Black-owned hair companies and brands to redesign a hair industry that has long ignored Black women and their hair. For Black hair care, the internet has become crucial in creating a communal hub for Black women—providing an unlimited space for spreading and exchanging information. Once the COVID-19 pandemic took over, the internet in the realm of

Black hair care became even more essential. The COVID-era lockdown resulted in the complete shutdown of places of business and commerce, including everywhere you would previously purchase your favourite hair care products.

Black hair care shops were not categorised as essential retail during this time, so even when high street supermarkets and health and beauty stores began to open up again, Black hair shops remained shut. The closure of hair shops, hairdressers and everything in between meant that the online space was really the only place for Black women to access the right level of care for their hair. The demand for online Black-owned retailers increased, Instagram and TikTok tutorials on hair care rose, and a lot more Black women began to experiment with DIY hair styles.

Word of mouth has long been the backbone of the hair care industry as opposed to traditional marketing. Many Black women will only visit a hairstylist they know personally or that has been recommended to them. Today, due to the rise of social media, the importance of traditional marketing has waned. With companies now able to tap directly into their desired demographics, social media has completely revolutionised marketing.

Hair straightening products, particularly chemical relaxers, have dominated the Black hair market ever since the industry began, but that's beginning to change. Since 2008, relaxer sales have steadily declined, and according to research conducted by Mintel in 2018, relaxers in the US make up 21% of the Black hair care market, which is down 15% since 2011.[20] This shift is due to the most recent iteration of the natural hair movement of the 2000s, with many Black women transitioning from relaxed hair to natural. Wellness has become an industry which has also contributed to this change. People are becoming more conscious of their way of life and the products they are consuming, from food to fitness to hair care.

Many Black women wear wigs, weaves and extensions as a means to protect their natural hair, which stays hidden underneath these hairstyles. These extensions aren't just straight, they come in infinite textures, colours, lengths and styles, providing versatility without compromising the health of the wearer's natural hair. This could also be a contributing factor to the decline in hair relaxers. In 2014, Mintel noted that 44% of Black women reported having a weave, wig or extensions in the past 12 months.[21] This aligns with responses I received in the survey I conducted, with 42.7% of Black women stating that their go-to hairstyles were wigs, weaves or some form of extensions. Wigs and weaves have always been around and worn from as early as the '70s, but in more recent years, Black women have popularised them, which has resulted in celebrities and influencers using wigs and weaves to change their looks on a regular basis. This has also led to the growth of the Black wig styling industry, with stylists now charging hundreds, if not thousands, of pounds to create high-quality, customised wigs.

When it comes to the many successful Black-owned hair care companies in the UK, Treasure Tress has done a phenomenal job in creating space for Black women and their hair. Founded by Jamelia Donaldson, Treasure Tress is the UK's first natural hair product discovery box. Customers subscribe to Treasure Tress and receive a box of various hair care items each month. Since its launch, the company has created a solid and growing natural hair community and has solidified itself as a successful Black-owned company. I spoke to founder

Jamelia Donaldson about all things hair and business.

INTERVIEW WITH JAMELIA DONALDSON, FOUNDER OF TREASURE TRESS

ZKS: Could you talk about your personal hair journey and how that contributed to your decision to start Treasure Tress?

JD: From a really young age, I just had a fascination with hair. I used to charge girls at school £5 to get a cool braid design on one section of their hair. After school, I would do my mum's friend's daughter's hair for £15, which wasn't actually a good price because it would take me 2 hours to do, but it was the start of something.

I got to the age of about 14 and decided that having my hair in its natural state made me look young. So I started straightening my hair and would do the same for my friends. I was doing that for a few years and I distinctly remember thinking, 'wow, my hair hasn't grown in length for a solid 10 years—why is that?' So I Googled, 'how to make Black hair grow,' which led me to this online community, the earliest version of a blog.

Then, YouTube started to get big. I remember watching videos of women talking about how they used to straighten their hair but now wear it in its natural state. That made me realise that I can make that transition. I wasn't ever allowed to use relaxer because my hair is naturally really fine. My mum always said, 'if you relax your hair it will drop out!' For that reason, I had the privilege of always being natural, but not really knowing what to do with [my hair] to make sure that it was healthy and make sure I could retain the length I wanted.

I started buying the products that the YouTubers were using, [...] and then mixing [them] with honey and making all these different concoctions and spray bottles with leave-in conditioner. My second year of university is when I stopped straightening my hair and started experimenting with my hair in its natural state. And it did look like a hot mess! I distinctly remember one of my friends saying, 'Jam, are you really going out with your hair like that?!'

In my third year of uni, I did an internship in New York. When I was in New York, I had access to all the hair products I wanted. And I noticed that there were lots of subscription boxes popping up for Black women. I remember wishing that we had a service like that in the UK. Long story short, I returned to the UK, did a corporate internship, that turned into a corporate graduate role, and while I was there I launched Treasure Tress.

ZKS: What is your ultimate vision for Treasure Tress?

JD: [To] transform the way that Black women discover and engage with products on multiple levels. It's about changing how they're marketed to, who is creating the marketing campaigns, what messages they are sharing, what models [they are casting] and what language they are using. [In terms of] formulation, what ingredients are included and how do we communicate what the benefits are? On an ownership level, a big part of my vision is to ensure that we own as many Black hair brands as possible because we are the consumers and we should also be the owners.

ZKS: You mentioned that you saw a subscription model in the US. Were there any challenges around getting people to buy into this idea in the UK?

JD: To my American peers, the concept made complete sense. To those in the UK, it was like, 'what? You want us to put money behind marketing to *Black women*?' This is still an issue we come across every single day. These brands have have all of this money and primarily target white women. The minute we want them to market to Black women, they don't have the budget to support it. Black women are the biggest consumers. They want Black women to consume their products but don't want to pay to acquire them as a customer. [...] Everyone wants a bit of the money that Black women spend, but they don't want to invest in the way that they do for other consumers, and that is the main challenge here in the UK. In America, they are very clued up on the power of the Black dollar, and so even if brands don't really believe in it, they'll pretend that they do. Whereas in the UK, they won't even bother investing in it until it's too late, and then they'll be scrambling for solutions.

ZKS: How has Treasure Tress and the brands you work with been impacted by events such as the COVID-19 pandemic?

JD: [2020 was a challenging] year, but some really good opportunities have come to the surface. The opportunity is the fact that we are a box that gets delivered directly to your front door. For half of the year, most people couldn't leave their house. So immediately, we had a huge surge in subscribers, which was brilliant. On the flip side, COVID did mean that a lot of manufacturing factories were shut down, so a lot of brands weren't producing products anymore. They were only producing hand sanitiser, or they were not producing the same quantities that they were before, or they were having logistical issues with shipping products from the US to the UK. Demand definitely went up, but that wasn't without logistical issues. We did see a sharp increase in sales and we worked hard to keep up with demand and stay sustainable. Overall, Covid was beneficial for us and [...] for customers, lockdown has made them rethink the way that they live and what they purchase.

ZKS: What do you think may be another game changer in the next few years and how do you see the industry evolving further?

JD: [W]ith regards to ownership, Black-owned brands are coming out thick and fast and the internet has provided us all with resources we can use to connect with consumers. [...]

We will continue to see improvements in ingredients because wellness is a huge focus right now and I don't think it's just a trend, it's a lifestyle change which is necessary for the planet. Representation [in marketing] is already changing (I hope). We'll shift [...] towards women of all complexions with kinkier, more coily hair types.

[What it means to 'be natural'] will change. As

of late, you wear your hair out, you wear braids, you wear hair out, and you wear braids again. But now, you wear wigs and weaves, but you're natural underneath. And I think that goes hand-in-hand with us as a Black community allowing Black women to express themselves however they want to. [...] As much as we will journey towards cleaner ingredients, it will be a personal journey for everyone, and we will grow in understanding of that. Just because someone continues to relax their hair doesn't mean that they care about their wellbeing less, it's just a different decision that they've made that works for their lifestyle. We will grow in understanding and empathy for everyone and their personal decisions on how they choose to do their hair.

7

THE SCIENCE OF
BLACK HAIR

In recent years, we have seen consumers put brands and organisations under more scrutiny in order to understand how they operate. How do they use customer data? How do they treat their workers? What impact are they having on the environment? What are they putting into the products they're selling?

Historically, consumers were not as societally conscious as they are today and up until recently, the hair care industry was no different. Previously, when we would go to the hairdressers, we would let them have their way with our hair without much question about the impact of the products used or what was being done to our hair—it is probably part of the reason why so many Black women, myself included, have hairdresser horror stories. Similarly, when we would purchase hair products, we would not research the ingredients in them. Today, things are different. Natural hair consumers have adopted a new approach that seeks to hold companies accountable and understand exactly what they are putting in their hair. But even with this shift in the psyche of the consumer, do we truly understand the effects that these products have on our hair and why? Do we even know what our hair is made of? In order to truly understand how best to care for our hair, we need to deepen our knowledge on the science behind it. Knowing how our hair is chemically structured and what ingredients make up our hair products will help us care for our hair in a way that enables it to thrive.

HAIR MYTHS

Before we get into the brilliant and hairy science of Black hair we must dispel a few myths. Myths in hair and beauty are a byproduct of topics we do not fully understand and when it comes to Black hair, there is a lot of misinformation (which is why reading this book is a great idea!). This section shall go into some of the most widely spread myths about natural Black hair, explaining how and why they are not true.

1. AFRO HAIR DOESN'T GROW.

All hair grows. On average, Afro hair can grow up to half an inch per month (so six inches in a year), but some of that length will be lost to dead ends that will need to be cut off. Curly hair can also mask growth due to shrinkage, which can be frustrating because you are unable to see the extent of developments in hair length. However, shrinkage is a sign of healthy, elastic hair, and we should remind ourselves that having long hair is not the be-all and end-all. We should instead prioritise hair health over hair length!

2. AFRO HAIR DOESN'T NEED TO BE WASHED OFTEN.

Due to the build-up of sebum, sweat, the hair products that we use and general exposure to the elements as we go about our day, it is important that we keep our hair and scalp regularly cleansed. Otherwise, the build-up will cause dryness. The general advice seems to be that Afro hair should be washed and conditioned once a week, and additionally moisturised in-between these washes to keep the hair supple.

3. OILING YOUR HAIR AND SCALP REGULARLY IS THE KEY TO KEEPING IT MOISTURISED.

Oil-based creams and conditioners often make the hair more pliable and easy to style and manipulate. Synthetic, petroleum-based oils are cheap and therefore used in many products e.g. baby oil. They provide skin and hair with softness and shine as they prevent moisture from escaping. The molecules of these oils are too big to penetrate our hair, which is why they form a film on the hair that can cause build-up. Oils are not true sources of moisture, which is why many Black women may still be prone to dryness and breakage no matter how much they try to cream or oil their hair. You need a moisture-based product combined with a protein-based product to keep your hair hydrated and thriving.

4. DIY PROTEIN TREATMENTS ARE BETTER THAN SHOP-BOUGHT ONES.

The majority of proteins are too big to penetrate the hair and so they sit on the surface of the hair instead. Protein treatments strengthen the hair but can also make it stiff if overused. This results in dry and brittle hair that can break easily, hence the importance of balancing protein with moisture. You may have come across people recommending protein treatments using ingredients such as yoghurt, egg and avocado. The problem with these sources of protein is that the molecules are too big—they will coat the hair but not get inside to strengthen it. To summarise, protein treatments are great in moderation and please experiment with DIY treatments at your own risk. I have heard one too many horror stories of women making a lovely homemade egg-protein treatment, applying it to their hair and mistakenly rinsing it out using water that is much too hot. The result? Scrambled egg on your scalp! A new hairstyle or a quick snack? I'll leave you to decide.

Coconut oil is one of the only oils with molecules small enough to penetrate the hair shaft and under the cuticle layers, preventing loss of protein. This makes it beneficial in hair care, especially before shampooing. When washing hair, we know that this causes the hair to expand and then contract, and when this happens too drastically, it can cause breakage. Applying coconut oil to your hair before shampooing it (called a pre-shampoo or pre-poo treatment) means that the coconut oil molecules bind to the hair, allowing less space for water to come in. This protects the hair from damage from drastic expansion and contraction.

STRUCTURE OF HAIR

When it comes to the hair on our heads, the scalp is the centre of all the activity. A healthy scalp is made up of a network of tissues, blood vessels and nerve endings. The hair itself is made up of proteins and grows from follicles in our scalp. Hair that is inside the follicle is alive but once it grows out of the scalp, its cells die. Although the hairs we can see on top of our heads (called the hair shaft) are dead, they respond to various stimuli, which we will explore in this chapter.

SCALP STRUCTURE

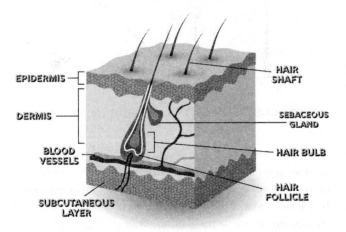

The hair shaft has a protective outer layer called the cuticle, which resembles tiles or scales along the hair shaft. The cuticle layer can open up or contract depending on what substances it comes into contact with. As the hair gets older and is exposed to friction, chemicals and over-styling, the cuticle layer becomes damaged and can cause the hair to break. Are you still following? Great!

HAIR TYPES

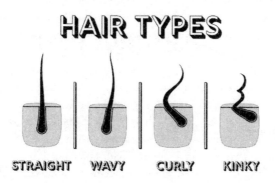

STRAIGHT   **WAVY**   **CURLY**   **KINKY**

The shape of our hair follicles determines what the texture of our hair will be. People with straight or wavy hair have hair follicles with a circular cross-section, and the hair grows straight out of the scalp, with no curling. Afro hair follicles are flatter and, if you were to cut through one horizontally, the cross section is uniquely kidney/oval-shaped, resulting in hair that grows up and around like a ribbon, with lots of twists and turns. People often assume that Afro hair is very tough or stronger than other hair types but this could not be further from the truth. For those with Afro hair, the hair shaft is actually more fragile than other hair types as it is more likely to tangle and break because of its curls. As a result, Afro hair needs greater care than straight or wavy hair, and relaxed Afro hair should be treated with even more care as the hair structure is weakened.

Hair porosity indicates the hair's ability to absorb water and other substances. Hair porosity will, therefore, depend on the condition of the cuticle layer and strength of the hair. Hair with open or damaged cuticles is said to have high porosity because it can't hold water well. It will take in lots of moisture but lose it just as easily, so it's important to use creams or oils on high porosity hair to lock in moisture and prevent the hair from drying out too easily. Hair with low porosity has cuticles that are closed and flat, which do not take in moisture or chemicals very well. With low porosity hair, products are more likely to sit on the hair shaft and cause a greasy build-up rather than be properly absorbed. Lighter, liquid-based moisturisers work well on low porosity hair. Natural Black hair tends to have lower porosity than Caucasian or Asian hair types.

If you are remotely familiar with hair and skin care, it is likely you have heard of the term sebum. Sebum is the natural oil of our hair and skin. The sebaceous gland is attached to the hair follicle and is responsible for producing sebum. Sebum conditions and lubricates our skin and scalp, preventing loss of moisture, and giving it a shiny look. Our production of sebum does not remain constant and can be impacted by factors such as hormones and our diet. Sebum can travel easily down straight hair but the shape of Afro hair, with all its kinks and curls, makes it harder for sebum to travel and spread. This makes Afro hair more likely to suffer from dryness.

Another cause of hair dryness is allowing sebum to build up in our hair and harden over time. Regularly oiling our scalp may sound like a good idea to keep our hair lubricated, but in reality, using lots of heavy oils and creams can obstruct sebum and cause further dryness and flakiness. Lighter oils such as coconut and jojoba are much better for our hair because rather than causing a blockage, their molecules are small enough to penetrate the hair shaft. Regularly cleansing our hair and scalp will remove any old oil and product build-up.

DIFFERENT FORMS:
RELAXED, TEXTURED, WET AND DRY.

Hair is made of proteins, primarily keratin, which is rich in the chemical element sulphur. I will use the term 'textured hair' to describe hair strands that have a non-straight form such as coils, waves or spirals. Textured hair has more disulphide bonds than straighter hair. What are disulphide bonds, I hear you ask? Disulphide bonding describes the process of two sulphur atoms forming a connection between each other. Because the keratin in our hair is full of sulphur, the sulphur atoms that are next to each other can form a strong chemical bond, which is what we call disulphide bonding (the prefix di- indicates that two atoms are bonded together). Disulphide bonds don't break easily but once the bond does break, it can't be reformed. One product that can break these strong bonds is chemical relaxer, which effectively removes the kinks in the hair and straightens it out. With the disulphide bonds broken, this weakens the hair structure, therefore relaxed hair usually requires more care than natural textured hair since it can be more prone to damage. Because the disulphide bonds are permanently broken, relaxed hair can't go back to its original natural state unless it grows out.

Hydrogen bonding is another important bond present in hair and is much weaker than disulphide bonding. When these bonds come into contact with water (or heat), they break down and form new bonds. This is how a lot of hairstyles work. For example, I wet my hair, breaking down the hydrogen bonds, and then braid it, which stretches the hair. As the hair dries, the hydrogen bonds reform. When I undo the braids, the curls are set in the new formation made by the braids, producing defined, zigzag curls. Hair can be styled in a similar way when it's dry, but given the lack of water, the hydrogen bonds don't fully break down, so the hair may not properly set into the new style. As a result, when doing styles like braid-outs on dry hair, they typically won't be as defined as when you're styling on wet hair.

When Black hair is healthy, it is elastic. If you stretch it and let go, it should return to its original curl length. Elasticity is an indicator of strength and allows hair to be moulded into different styles, otherwise, it would just break. Wet hair is more elastic than dry hair, which is why it's always best to comb and detangle hair when damp, to reduce the risk of breakage.

Shrinkage is a characteristic of textured hair and describes the way that wet hair springs back into shape as it dries. By staying coily rather than stretched, the hair appears to be much shorter in length and this is a particular pain point for Black women in a world where long hair is praised.

A lot of Black hair products are protein-rich in order to rebuild Black hair that may have been damaged by chemical relaxers or too much heat. Most hair breakage is the result of too many protein-rich products and not enough moisture, or over-styling the hair.

In addition to shrinking and breaking, hair can also shed. The difference between breakage and shedding is that breakage is a response to something that has been done to the hair and can be solved by changing your styling technique or assessing how much moisture or protein your hair needs. Shedding, on the other hand, occurs naturally as part of the hair growth cycle that each individual hair goes through, where it falls from the scalp. Shedding is normal, however, if you notice your hair shedding more than usual, or experience unexpected hair loss, then it may be useful to see a trichologist to understand if any underlying issues are causing this.

INTERVIEW WITH TRICHOLOGIST EBUNI AJIDUAH

A trichologist is a specialist who focuses on the hair and scalp, understanding the diseases and conditions relating to those two areas. Despite their importance in the hair and skin world, the role of a trichologist is not as well known as it should be amongst the general public. Ebuni Ajiduah is a trichologist based in the UK who focuses on Black hair and scalps. I got the chance to speak with Ebuni Ajiduah about her career and Black hair care.

ZKS: What is trichology and when should someone consider seeing a trichologist?

EA: Trichology is the study of the hair and scalp. It sits somewhere between hairdressing and dermatology but we mostly focus on hair loss and scalp disorders. Trichologists are the people you come and see if you're having any issues with your hair and scalp; chronic dryness, hair loss, anything like that. If you are concerned about your hair but can't pinpoint the issue or you're not able to solve it yourself, that's when you might need to see a trichologist.

ZKS: How did you get into trichology?

EA: I always loved doing hair. At school, I would do my friends' hair and then I started to do their parents' hair too. I started a career in science teaching but realised that it wasn't for me. I really wanted to focus on hair again so I quit teaching and formally became a hairdresser. In the process of doing this, I started seeing a lot of people with hair loss, but in the salon, we weren't really taught about how to deal with hair loss or what the causes are. I came across lots of people with different hair conditions and I felt like I didn't have the tools, or even the words, to explain to them what was happening to their hair and where they needed to go to get help, advice or treatment.

I can't remember how I came across trichology but I remember thinking, 'science and hair? I get to mix the two? Perfect.' I was sold. At the time I was living in Dubai, and I couldn't find anywhere local to me to begin studying. When I came back to London, I found an online course with a training facility in Manchester. And that's when I decided to pursue trichology.

ZKS: What has been your experience of studying and practising trichology?

EA: The whole way through my course, with every condition I learnt about, I had to ask 'but what about Black people? What about Afro hair? How would this look on Black skin?' The symptoms of a condition would say, 'it shows redness,' or 'the scalp would change in this way,' and I would think, 'that doesn't happen to my scalp,' or 'my skin wouldn't react in this way.'

From the beginning, I thought more needed to be done in this area to support Black women. The little information that was available about Black women was focused on self-inflicted conditions such as traction alopecia through doing very tight hairstyles that damage our hair. I was like, 'yeah but it can't all just be this? What else is going on?'

I found it difficult, but getting to practice is one of the most rewarding things I've done. There is a lack of Black trichologists in general, and I feel like Black women aren't listened to, especially when it comes to health care. Being able to provide a service where I can listen to and help them, and seeing the relief on their faces after has been so rewarding. They're like, 'I've known there was something wrong and finally I have the answer to what I've been searching for.'

ZKS: What are the main hair conditions that you have seen Black women, in particular, suffer with?

EA: When people talk about hair loss they always use the term alopecia. Alopecia just means hair loss. So if you tell me that you have alopecia, you haven't told me anything. I know your hair is falling out, but I don't know why. There's specific names for different types of alopecia, which have their own associated treatment. There's a type of scarring alopecia, called CCCA, which is when something goes wrong in the hair growth process and the follicle becomes so scarred and inflamed it stops producing hairs completely. When Instagram first came out, I would see a lot of stylists doing braiding styles to cover hair loss in the middle of the scalp. This used to be called hot comb alopecia because it was thought that the cause was heat styling damaging the centre of the scalp. It's something that is happening to Black women at an alarming rate and it's not being taken as seriously as it needs to be. I would say around 80–90% of Black women I see with this condition have gone to their GP to ask for help and they're told that, 'it's just hair loss, it doesn't really matter, you should just accept it.' But they can lose 50% of their hair or more through this condition, which can be difficult when so many Black people take pride in their hair. It can be really heartbreaking, especially when you are told that the issue is your own fault.

The other issues I see are mostly scalp issues. A dry, flaky scalp is a really common one and is exacerbated by the practices that we have. When everyone used to use relaxers, we were told that our hair doesn't like water because otherwise the relaxed hair would not stay straight. That has transpired in the natural hair scene as well, so we're not used to washing our hair as frequently as we should. All of that leads to a build-up of bacteria and oils on our scalp, which can worsen certain conditions. Rather than thinking about what additional oils or products you could apply to your hair to remove the flakiness, you should think about washing your hair more often and seeing if that helps. Some products will make the symptoms subside temporarily but then it may come back with a vengeance. It's a vicious cycle of having temporary relief and continuing to use the products, but not fixing the underlying issue.

ZKS: Are you seeing more Black women beginning to understand their hair on a deeper level than before? How do you think things will improve in the future?

EA: At the beginning of my journey, I got disheartened. I realised how mammoth my task was. When I finished my trichology class, I realised that everything I knew about hair was wrong. Nothing made sense. I felt like we'd been going backwards all this time. Online communities have been so crucial to help spread knowledge. Even me, in my little corner of the world on social media, I'm just putting out information and people manage to find me and learn more about hair issues. There's loads of us out there now who are trying to get people's attention and debunking myths.

We shouldn't underestimate the power of the internet and social media. With the rise of Black social media influencers, we're starting to see more diversity in content. There's also now a generation of women who have relaxed their hair and now gone back to natural. When they decide to have children, they might decide that their children are never going to see a relaxant in their life. This is literally breaking generational practices of relaxing Black girls' hair, and this could prevent a whole generation of women from experiencing the trauma that many of us did.

HAIR PRODUCTS

We all have that one subject or topic that we learnt in school that, upon reflection, has materialised into the most pointless use of our time. I am here to tell you that out of all those subjects, chemistry is NOT one of them. That's right folks, next up, we will be looking at pH and its importance in relation to hair care. This is going to be a quick, crash course, so for a deep dive into some of the topics covered in this chapter, I recommend reading *The Science of Black Hair* by Audrey Davis-Sivasothy.

The pH of certain products can impact our hair in huge ways—both good and bad. pH stands for 'potential for hydrogen'.[1] pH measures the concentration of hydrogen ions in a solution in relation to distilled water (also known as 'pure' water).

The pH scale ranges from 0 to 14, with distilled water

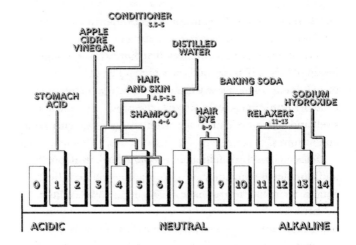

sitting at the middle of the scale with a pH of 7, which we call neutral. A solution with a pH of below 7 is acidic and has a higher concentration of hydrogen ions than water. A pH of above 7 means that the solution is alkaline, or basic.

The pH scale is logarithmic, which means that a step up or down the scale represents a 10 times change in hydrogen ions. For example, pH 5 is 10 times more acidic than pH 6, and 100 times more acidic than pH 7. This is important as a small change in pH can have a very big impact on our hair.

Hair and skin are slightly acidic with a pH of around 4.5–5.5. The effect of acidic substances on our hair makes the cuticle layers close up and lie flat against the surface of the hair shaft. This makes hair smoother and gives it a shinier look because when the cuticles contract in this way, they reflect light better, as well as lock in moisture more effectively.

Substances that are alkaline make the hair cuticle layers open up and cause the hair shaft to soften and swell. In this state, the hair cannot hold moisture well and the result is dry, dull hair. Because water is more alkaline than hair, it has this effect on hair unless something is added to the hair to lower its pH and make the cuticle go back to its normal state.

When exposed to substances that are extremely high or low in pH level, hair can become very damaged. Strong acids, of pH 2 and below, cause the hair to contract so much that it becomes brittle and breaks. Strong bases, of pH 13 and above, swell and soften the hair to the point where it becomes weak and dissolves.

Shampoos and conditioners regulate the pH of our hair and can therefore maintain or improve the quality of the hair cuticle. Shampoos tend to have a pH of 4–6, with conditioners deliberately having a lower pH of around 3.5–5. Conditioners being more acidic than shampoos means that once your hair is cleansed, conditioning it will close the cuticles, preventing damage and loss of moisture. Shampoos and conditioners from the same product range will be formulated to achieve the right pH balance when used together, but products from different ranges and brands may differ in their pH levels. It may be useful to buy pH strips, also known as litmus paper, for an easy way to test the pH of a skin or hair product. This can help you check how your shampoos and conditioners balance pH and what products may work best together for your hair.

Let's dig a bit deeper into shampoos and conditioners since they are the foundation of good hair care. Shampoos hydrate the hair and cleanse it by removing any dirt and product build-up. Regularly shampooing and conditioning hair restores it of moisture, which is particularly important for Afro-textured hair. Many shampoos include chemicals called sulphates, which are strong detergents. They do a great job at stripping hair of dirt, but they also remove the hair's natural oils. Common sulphate-based ingredients found in shampoos are ammonium lauryl/laureth sulphate (ALS) and sodium lauryl/laureth sulphate (SLS). With Afro-textured hair, these natural oils already struggle to travel along the length of the curls and thus shampoos containing sulphates can cause hair to feel dry and coarse. To prevent the hair from fully drying out, it's important to properly condition it after shapooing. Most shampoo brands still include sulphates because of their effectiveness at stripping the hair of any build-up. However, more recently there has been a rise in sulphate-free (or specifically ALS- and SLS-free) products that cleanse the scalp more lightly, therefore helping it to retain its natural oils better. Personally, I like to use a sulphate-based shampoo every now and again to give my hair a deep cleanse and sulphate-free shampoo on a more regular basis. Next time you're shopping for shampoo, check the ingredients for sulphates and take time to explore which shampoo (or combination of shampoos) may work for you.

Conditioning our hair after shampooing and rinsing it is arguably the most important part of the hair care routine. Conditioners stick to the hair cuticles and restore moisture that is lost through shampooing, therefore maintaining the protein/moisture balance in our hair. Conditioners keep our hair strong but soft and shiny. A lot of conditioning products contain ingredients that sebum is made up of, such as glycerine and cholesterol. These products aim to do a similar job to the natural sebum in our hair, keeping the hair from losing moisture.

When reading the ingredients on hair products, the ingredients are listed in order of highest concentration in the product to lowest.[2] Moisturisers should always have water or aqua as the first ingredient in the list, which makes sense since the primary job of a moisturiser is to hydrate the hair. Ingredients such as petrolatum, mineral oil, waxes and silicones are often found in moisturisers. They coat the hair and give it a shiny look, but can build up and actually block any moisture from entering or leaving the hair and scalp. These substances can retain moisture well, but stop any more moisture from entering the hair, which can ultimately lead to dryness. The build-up of these products can often be difficult to remove, requiring extra cleansing. When looking for moisturisers, you may wish to choose one which doesn't contain many of the above ingredients, or contains them in small concentrations (so should be listed towards the end of the ingredients list on the product label).

Hair relaxers are a popular hair product due to their ability to permanently straighten Afro-textured hair. Relaxers come in the form of a thick white cream that is lathered onto the hair. It works by breaking down the strong disulphide bonds in our hair, altering the structure of the hair. Once applied, relaxers should be left on the head for about 15 minutes before being thoroughly rinsed out with warm water and washed with a neutralising shampoo to get the hair's pH back down to normal. Use of hair relaxers has been a controversial topic for a number of years because of the chemicals that relaxers contain and the negative effects that they can have on hair. Lye and caustic soda are alternative names for the chemical sodium hydroxide, which is the main component of hair relaxers. Sodium hydroxide is extremely alkaline; we're talking pH 14. This chemical is used in strong cleaning products such as drain unblockers because it's so corrosive. If left on the hair for too long, it will melt away the protective hair cuticle layers and burn the scalp. This weakens the hair structure and ultimately thins the hair. There are also no-lye relaxers, which substitute sodium hydroxide with weaker chemicals, such as calcium hydroxide, and are less harsh on the scalp than sodium hydroxide. However, these substitutes can often dry out the hair more so may not necessarily be 'better' for your hair.

Sodium hydroxide, or caustic soda, is corrosive and when

it comes into contact with the scalp, it can cause burning and scabbing. The chemical toxins in hair relaxers can then be absorbed through the scalp tissue, ultimately entering the bloodstream. Relaxers are so strong that even being around relaxers for too long can ultimately cause lung damage through inhalation. For women who relax their hair frequently over a long period, this can have long-term health effects on the body. Relaxers often contain parabens and phthalates. Parabens are chemicals that can disrupt the body's hormone balance and have been linked to cancer, weight gain and reduced muscle mass. Phthalates are chemicals that make plastics more flexible and durable and they are found everywhere—from cleaning products to plastic packaging to perfume.[3] Phthalates are linked to breast and ovarian cancer as well as early menopause. The National Institute of Environmental Health Sciences released a study reporting that women who use chemical hair straighteners every five to eight weeks were about 30% more likely to develop breast cancer than those who don't.[4]

It's not uncommon for Black women to have their hair relaxed from as young as five years old. You can't help but wonder whether this would be allowed if hair relaxers were targeted at and used by white people. Given the potential long-lasting effects of relaxers on women who use them for multiple years of their lives, it makes me question why these products are not more regulated.

HAIR TYPES

For a long time, Black people didn't have access to the information needed to properly care for their hair. Luckily, that has changed, and we have more stylists and experts on hand to provide support. It's great that there are professionals to turn to, but it's also important that Black women understand their

HAIR TYPES

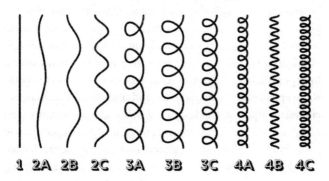

1 2A 2B 2C 3A 3B 3C 4A 4B 4C

own hair to ensure that it's staying as healthy as it can be. A common way for Black women to do this is by using the Andre Walker Hair Typing System. Walker was Oprah Winfrey's personal hairstylist. The hair typing system was created by him in the 1990s to promote his range of hair products and it soon became a popular way of determining hair type.

The idea is that by using Walker's simple chart you can identify your hair type and take the first step towards understanding your hair needs. The chart starts with Type 1, which is straight hair, and as you move down the chart, the hair gets curlier. Type 2 hair is wavy, Type 3 hair is curly and the last type, Type 4, is kinky. On the chart, letters from A–C are placed next to the numbers, which determine how coily the hair is. Therefore, Type 4C hair is more coiled than Type 4A hair.

The chart, whilst a relatively useful categorisation method, does not represent all hair types. Hair and its texture are unique and complex things and cannot be embodied by a chart with four main categories. This is a good foundation, however, it's not the full picture. I have seen countless articles about 'the best products for 4C hair', but the product that someone may require doesn't just depend on what their curls look like. It depends on their moisture levels, the state of their hair cuticles and any potential hair damage. Some of these recommendations and popular products for certain hair types may not work for you, and that's totally fine. There are so many variables when it comes to hair and there isn't one set method that will work for everyone. The hair typing system also fails to take into consideration that many people have a variety of hair types growing from their scalp. Perhaps most worrying is that this hair chart associates straight hair with being primary, Type 1 hair, leaving everything else in relation to Type 1 as a divergence from the standard.

8
WHO DID YOUR HAIR? THE WORLD OF HAIRSTYLING

Afro hair requires a very particular level of care in comparison to other hair types due to its fragility and unique structure. Throughout time, hair styling has been an integral part of Black and African culture. Although we no longer style our hair depending on our position and status within society, hair is still used as a way to express ourselves. For example, when I reflect on how I decide to style my hair, it tends to be influenced by how I'm feeling. If I'm in the mood to stand out and feel bold, I'll let my hair loose and wear my afro out. If I feel like going for something a bit more subtle and understated, I might slick my hair back into a bun. For a style that feels free and flowing, I might go for braid extensions. When considering the versatility of Afro hair, it is no surprise that Black women change their hairstyles more regularly than any other group. Just walking into a local Black hair shop opens your eyes to a world of possibilities. Gels, beads, clips, extensions, wigs, rollers, combs, not to mention the endless shelves of products.

For many Black women, hair styling starts at home. Your mum commands you to sit down so that she can comb out your hair and grease it. You're taken to your aunt's house so that she can put your hair into cornrows or braids. These experiences are social, informal and intimate. As we get older, the hair styling process moves from the home into the Black hair salon.

In the '40s and '50s, there was an influx of Black people moving to Britain, so the demand for Black hair care was high. However, most existing salons would not cater to Afro-textured hair. At the time, Afro hair was not included in standard hairdressing courses and qualifications. This remains largely unchanged today, with those wishing to study Afro hair having to pay an additional fee to do so. It was only in 2021 that the National Occupational Standards for hairdressing officially included Afro-textured hair as a styling practice, meaning that all hairdressers are required to learn how to style Black hair.

Carmen Maingot and Winifred Atwell are understood to have potentially opened up two of the first Black hair salons in the UK. Maingot, who was one of the founders of Notting Hill Carnival, opened her salon in 1955.[1] Her salon was based in South Kensington and specialised in straightening hair. Atwell opened her salon in 1957 in Brixton after her successful music career.[2] In her salon, Atwell also offered hair straightening services and taught women how to style Black hair.

A couple of decades later in the '70s, Winston Isaacs founded the Splinters hair salon, which is documented as the first high-end salon for Afro-textured hair. Located in the West End of London, Splinters attracted prestigious clientele from across the world, including celebrities.

In 2017, a study by the Hair and Beauty Industry Authority showed that there are 35,704 registered salons in the UK, but only 302 of them are Afro hair salons.[3] I imagine the majority of these are found in London. Of course, a lot of Afro hair stylists may not be affiliated with a salon, so are not included in this number, but this raises the question of why nearly all salons don't cater to Black hair.

The Black hair salon is often a safe space for women who

use its services. These environments are usually organically created, evolving from the Black home itself and for many Black women, these spaces remind them of home. This authentic, communal feel, whilst generally positive, perhaps stems from the fact that some Black hairstylists and salons are not professionally trained. This could be part of the reason why a considerable amount of Black women have at least one hair salon horror story. Combining that with the preconceptions people have regarding Black businesses providing subpar customer service, some Black women do not trust Black hair salons with their hair care.

The Black women who took my survey shared some of their not-so-nice experiences at the Black hair salon.

'Being told my hair was too dense to work with by hairdressers from a young age made me feel there was something wrong with me.'

'A hairdresser once told me that my hair was nothing but frizz. I am still trying to recover from that!'

'When I was a young child my Mum struggled with my hair saying I had bad hair, felt like my hair wasn't nice, tried all the chemicals from secondary school, curly perm, relaxers, braids until becoming a hairdresser and now a technical educator.'

At the start of this book, I detailed my own memories of sitting at home with my mother styling my hair. Interestingly, the crux of Black hair styling seems to be returning back home. Today our hairstylists are not always found in registered salons, but rather in the Black girl who lives down the road who is good at doing braids, or the other Black girl who is a friend of a friend and makes wigs in her bedroom. A number of hairstylists have grown booming businesses through promoting their services on social media platforms. Rather than paying for a chair in a salon with limited opening hours, these stylists open up their homes all day, everyday, for their clients, or have mobile businesses where they travel to their client's location to do their hair.

This organic style of entrepreneurship is not new and is something that Black women have been doing for years. Now, thanks to social media, the ability for Black women to have thriving hair businesses from the comfort of their own home has reached new heights. The internet has helped to connect hairstylists to clients quickly and easily. Online platforms such as FroHub have enabled this by providing a booking system for Afro hairstylists. Founded by Rahel Tesfai after feeling as though her hair was not being catered to on the high street, FroHub helps customers to discover local Afro hairstylists who specialise in Black hair. For the hair stylists, Frohub is another way for them to grow their customer base and not have to rely so heavily on word of mouth or their social media platforms. For customers, they can find stylists for particular hairstyles and become part of the FroHub community for hair guidance and information.

INTERVIEW WITH HAIR STYLIST
CHARLOTTE MENSAH

Several Black hairstylists who made their mark on the UK hair industry began their career journeys at Winston Isaacs's salon, Splinters, one of them being the legendary Charlotte Mensah.

Mensah came from humble beginnings but made a name for herself as a skilled hairstylist. Eventually she opened up her own salon, Hair Lounge, and launched her own hair products—the award-winning Manketti Oil hair range. In 2018, Mensah would become the first Black woman to be inducted into the British Hairdressing Awards Hall of Fame. Now, with over thirty years of experience, Mensah is one of the leading figures in the Black British hair industry. In 2020 she released her first book, *Good Hair*, which delves into all things Black hair styling and aims to empower people to embrace their hair. I spoke to Charlotte Mensah about her journey in the hair industry, entrepreneurship, the natural hair movement and more.

ZKS: What has fueled your passion for hair styling and how would you describe your personal journey with your hair?

CM: I refer to myself firstly as a natural hair care specialist, which informs how I think about hair. I'm 50 now, and I've consciously lived through a number of eras of what I'd call 'Black hair'. We've gone from kinks to curly perms, relaxers to box braids, to weaves and wigs and now to more natural styles. If I'm honest, I have enjoyed every minute of it. The main reason why I believe I'm so successful is because I put the care of my client's hair first. There's no wrong way to wear your hair; wear it proud, wear it loud, but care for it first. My experience in the industry has greatly taught me that, and I have proactively sought to educate the masses on this. For instance, I had a column in the UK Black hair magazine called *Natural Fix* over 15 years ago, where I'd do a number of natural hairstyles on models detailing the look and why these styles were important to preserving your hair. At present, I'm on a natural hair growth journey, wearing braids as a protective style to stimulate hair growth. Watch this space!

ZKS: Why did you start up Hair Lounge and at the time, what was your vision for the business? What has been the highlight of your career journey?

CM: I was very much at a crossroads in my professional career. I had completed an apprenticeship at Splinters (the then Mecca of Black hair) 10 years prior and had spent the years since improving my craft. [...] I had built up quite a solid client base, so this felt like the natural next step. I knew I had the talent, skill and the business acumen to make it work but like all things in life, I needed a helping hand. The Princes' Trust was just that, providing a grant and mentorship that helped me devise a business plan that would still inform what I do today. My vision was to create a world-class hair care experience that made clients not only love their hair but cherish the time and experience they spent in my salon... There have been many highlights, but perhaps the most poignant was being inducted into the British Hairdressing Hall of Fame in 2018. It was quite literally the exemplification of my personal goal and it was a particularly sentimental moment—I received that award in the very hotel my father worked in as a kitchen porter when he first came to the UK. A journey to say the least.

ZKS: How did you start up the Manketti Oil Hair range and why Manketti oil?

CM: We launched in March 2016. Manketti was a

luxury product that sought to be seen in a noisy world. I had a job out in Serengeti and got the most amazing full-body massage. I had to investigate and soon became acquainted with the wonderful world of the Manketti nut.

My drive to build this product range was born out of a desire to [help] my clients and [everyone with] curly-haired textures. It's a known fact that finding Afro hair products that meet the needs of women in formulation, performance, smell and of course, in luxury, is a big challenge.

We are still very much in our infancy, but I'm thankful for the universal acclaim we received since inception. [...] We initially launched with three products; the shampoo, conditioner and oil. We have since added a finishing mist, [a] paddle brush, pomade and a candle for the home. The goal is to continue expanding the brand as our customers' needs become more apparent. Never doing too much, but enough to keep people engaged and above all, supported in their hair care journey. As a Ghanaian, I have always felt it was super important to create a strong brand presence back home, so getting stocked in some of the bigger hair salons has been imperative. I'm currently exploring avenues for a permanent physical presence in Accra. To add to that, America has and continues to be the place to be for all things curly hair; if you're not there, you're not doing something right! That's the next goal.

ZKS: You have three decades of experience in the Afro hair industry. How do you feel the industry has evolved over the years and what are the key events that contributed to this?

CM: I'm very proud to say that today's hairdressing is not just about chemical treatments as it was when I started. I hate the concept of trends, but I can't deny we're in a unique time where we can see natural hairstyles popularised everywhere in society, and as a result, clients can now see themselves rocking these styles. New technology in Afro hairdressing has brought a new degree of professionalism to the career, with people not only wanting styles that look good but ones that put the health of their hair first. You look at all the leading producers of hair care apparatus, Dyson, GHD etc. there all looking at the Afro and textured hair market and understanding that they need to make products that cater to these hair types. I think it's a combination of visual representation, easily accessible information and technology catered towards our hair types that have generally improved peoples' perceptions around 'good hair'.

ZKS: How do you feel about the knowledge gap in Black natural hair styling?

CM: As mentioned earlier, we need to address this head-on and in the most formal of manners. To put it simply, Afro hair doesn't get the respect it deserves. If a Black girl does an apprenticeship in hairstyling, she will most certainly learn how to create and work on European hairstyles, even if she has no desire of working on European hair. It should work both ways. Some of the biggest actors, musicians and pioneers of pop culture are Black or of Black descent. If we think it makes sense for these people to be the faces in our society, then it makes sense that people know how to recreate the styles they wear. I recently joined the National Apprenticeship Board for hair and I'm looking to shake the room up as far as possible. I'm optimistic, they reached out to me so there's a desire to make this change.

ZKS: When it comes to hair care what do you see as the biggest challenges/misconceptions that Black women have?

CM: One, that natural hair is strong. Natural hair looks strong, which is why so many people abuse it with rough treatment. In reality, Black hair is fragile and needs to be treated with the gentlest of care in order for it to flourish. Paddle brushes, wide-tooth combs and natural ingredients are the best tools and products for natural hair. Low manipulation and protective styles help to retain length because constant grooming can be too much for some hair types, especially 4C.

Two, that natural hair doesn't grow. Afro hair in its natural state tends to shrink up, preventing you from seeing its real length. You can grow your hair as long as it's destined to be. [...] Your hair is growing, but you may not be retaining the length due to chemical abuse, excess heat styling and a general lack of proper care.

Three, that split ends can be repaired with products. Once the hair has split it cannot be repaired. Some products advertise repair and temporary mends. The only way to get rid of split ends is to trim them every 6–8 weeks.

Four, that silk scarfs and silk pillowcases aren't necessary. Cotton scarves and pillowcases can cause friction on the already naturally porous textured hair.

However, wrapping your hair in a silk scarf will help to promote healthier and shinier hair. They help to keep your hair soft, moisturised and free of tangles.

COMMON HAIRSTYLES

When it comes to hairstyles, no one does them like Black women (if you don't agree, argue with yourself). The myriad of hairstyles that Black women create and re-design are gorgeously complex art forms. It would be impossible for me to list every single hairstyle created and worn by Black women, but I shall go into some of the most well-known Black hair styles. See pages 119-126 for photographic images of these styles.

AFRO

The afro hairstyle is achieved by combing out nautral Afro hair to form a full, round shape. As we have previously explored, this style was popularised around the '60s and '70s and is often associated with the civil rights movement and the Black Panther Party. Prior to this, many Black people would straighten their hair in order to assimilate into society.

Combing Afro-textured hair when it is completely dry can cause it to break, and so it's important to be gentle when combing hair out into an afro and avoid using a very thin-toothed comb. Minimal product should be applied to the hair because too much product will weigh the hair down and the afro won't be able to stand up. Split the hair into sections and comb through each section until it is detangled, starting from the ends up to the scalp. Slowly comb your way up to the scalp, only moving further up once the hair feels fully combed out.

WASH-AND-GO

The clue is in the name. You quite literally wash your hair, apply some product (usually a leave-in conditioner and some styling product such as a curl defining cream) and then go about your day. There is no further manipulation and so this style displays your hair's natural curl pattern. Wash-and-gos can be left out or tied in different ways to produce varying looks.

It's important to keep the hair moisturised when doing a wash-and-go, otherwise the hair can become very dry. Wash-and-gos can usually last a couple of days (or three or four if you're lucky) until you need to revive your curls again.

BLOWOUT

A blowout is when the hair is blow-dried and combed out, which achieves a smooth, soft look. The heat of the hair dryer stretches out the natural curls. Hair should be slightly damp when blow-drying, either from being washed beforehand, or, at the very least, spritzed with water to be slightly damp. Minimal product should be applied to the hair when blowing it out—just a leave-in conditioner and some type of heat protectant would be sufficient.

I find that using a hair dryer with a comb attachment is the easiest way of blowing out my hair. If you don't have a comb attachment, you can use a regular hair dryer and paddle brush or wide-toothed comb to comb through the hair while you're drying it. When blowing out the hair, split it into sections and start from the ends, ensuring that the hair is dried and detangled before making your way up to the scalp.

SILK PRESS

A silk press describes the process of straightening hair with heat using a hot comb and/or flat iron. The hot comb has been around since the 1870s, and it grew in popularity amongst Black people in the early 1900s due to Madame CJ Walker. A silk press quite literally means pressing the hair with heat until it is silky. This is a form of stretching hair, since the natural curls are ironed out due to the high levels of heat used.

To achieve a perfect silk press, hair should be properly cleansed to remove any product build-up. Deep conditioning the hair will close the hair cuticles and make the silk press smooth and shiny. Then, you should blow out the hair so that it is dry and stretched before pressing it with heat straighteners. Be sure to use a heat protectant product when straightening hair in this way to prevent heat damage.

Silk presses are temporary. If you want to maintain your silk press for as long as possible, you will need to avoid any form of moisture, from rain to your own sweat! Moisture will cause the silk press to lose it's straightness and go back to the natural curls. This applies to any style where you are using heat, such as a blowout.

RELAXED HAIR

Applying chemical hair relaxer permanently straightens one's hair by altering its natural curl texture. Relaxing hair is the most effective way of straightening hair; however, there is a higher risk of damage if not applied properly. It may be best for a professional to relax your hair for you instead of doing it yourself.

When relaxing hair yourself, it's important to follow the instructions provided with the product. Most will advise you to shampoo and deep condition your hair a few days before relaxing it. When relaxing hair for the first time, the relaxer should be applied to the whole hair shaft but not the scalp. When re-relaxing the hair, care should be taken to only apply the relaxer to the roots where there is new hair growth. Applying a relaxer to already relaxed hair could cause excess thinness and breakage. The relaxer should stay on the hair for about 15 minutes before being fully washed out.

Relaxers have been incredibly popular amongst Black women for the best part of a century; however, in recent years we are seeing its popularity decline and more women transition to natural hair and adopt more protective styles such as wigs and weaves.

TWISTS

To obtain twists, the hair is divided into sections. Each section should be combed through and split into two strands of hair which are then twisted around one another and downwards. Keep twisting all the way to the very ends of the hair to prevent the twist from unravelling. Some people may wish to use a holding gel or oil on the ends of the twists or throughout the hair to keep the twists neat and smooth. Twisting hair is a form of stretching. Undoing the twists and wearing them out produces another style called a 'twist-out'. Extensions can be used to produce longer twists by weaving additional hair in from the scalp.

BRAIDS/PLAITS

Braids, also known as plaits, are similar to twists, however, instead of two strands of hair, each section is split into three. These strands of hair are woven around one another in the following way: the right strand is brought to the middle of the other two strands. The left strand is then brought into the middle of those strands. The new right hand strand is then brought into the middle of the other two strands, etc. For a more comprehensive description and tutorial, which will make more sense than this, please explore the internet. This is another form of stretching and can also be undone and worn out as a 'braid-out' hairstyle. Due to the differing patterns, a twist-out and a braid-out will produce different outcomes. Hair can be braided with or without hair extensions.

BANTU KNOTS

Bantu knots are created by parting the hair into sections. Each section is twisted (or braided) and then wrapped around itself to form a knot on the scalp. The hairstyle gets its name from the Bantu people, who are reported to have created and popularised the style. The Bantu people represent over 300 ethnic groups covering a large region of central, south and southeast Africa who spoke the Bantu language.[4]

Similar to a twist-out and braid-out, Bantu knots can be undone to produce curls that can be worn out.

CANEROWS/CORNROWS

Canerows, or cornrows, are very similar to braids but instead of the braids hanging from the scalp, canerows are braided flat and along the scalp. Canerows have been used to create intricate hair designs for centuries. Hair should be combed and detangled prior to canerowing to ensure it doesn't get knotted in the process.

For a clear and easy description of how to canerow, please check out our good friend, the internet. As someone who has only recently learned to canerow, I'm not the best person to be providing guidance on the perfect technique. In short, canerows are started in a similar way to braiding hair. The hair should be parted based on how you want the canerow to look. Then, three small strands should be taken from the top of this section, and started off like a regular braid. Instead of weaving those individual strands together until the end, with each weave, more hair should be picked up from the section and added to each of the strands. This essentially 'ties' the braid to the scalp, forming a canerow that runs across the section that you parted.

LOCKS

Locks, also known as dreadlocks, are achieved by leaving hair to become matted on its own. Locks created in this way are often called 'freeform' locks to highlight the fact that they have been made naturally with minimal manipulation. Locks can be formed using other methods, which require more manipulation, including techniques such as braiding, twisting and adding extensions.

The origin of dreadlocks is complicated and eclectic, and has been subject of much debate over the years. The earliest written reference of locks is found in Hindu texts dating back to 1500 BC.[5] There is archaeological evidence of locks in the mummified remains of ancient Egyptians as well as the pre-Colombian Incan civilisation in Peru. In certain cultures in South Asia and the Middle East, allowing uncombed hair to form into matted locks is a symbol of the rejection of materialism and vanity.[6] In parts of Africa, locks are associated with strength and only worn by warriors like the Fula and Wolof people of West Africa and the Maasai and Kikuyu tribes of Kenya.[7] Locks are also commonly associated with

Rastafarianism and Jamaican culture. Many Rastafarians believe that hair is sacred and spiritual, hence they grow it out and avoid cutting and manipulating it.

WIGS/WEAVES

Wigs, weaves and extensions have been around for a long time, existing in numerous cultures and nations from Africa to Europe. Reports and traces of adding artificial hair onto your own hair can be found dating back to 5000 BC and it is not unreasonable to think that this practice could have existed even before that. In the 20th century, wig and weave wearing gained specific popularity amongst Black women in the last few decades.

Weave refers to additional hair (human or artificial) that is integrated with one's own hair, adding more length or volume. Hair weaves can be applied in a myriad of ways, two of the most common being glued or sewn in. In May 1951, Louisiana-born Christina Jenkins would file a patent for what she described as, 'permanently attaching commercial hair to live hair.'[8] Jenkins would call the technique the 'Hair-Weeve'. At the time, it was common practice for women to apply their weaves by pinning the artificial hair onto their natural hair with hair pins and clips, which would lead to a clunky, visibly unnatural look. Jenkins's technique would change the game and cause artificial hair to be attached more seamlessly than was previously possible. Jenkins's process consisted of three chords and a weaving frame allowing the weave to attach easily.[9] Jenkins's technique is known as the 'sew-in'.

A wig, also known as a wig cap, refers to a head covering with human or artificial hair attached. Whilst there are similarities between a wig and a weave, the main difference lies in the fact that the weave process consists of hair weft extensions instead of a full head covering/cap of hair.

Both wigs and weaves have become far more versatile, particularly in comparison to those that were around when Jenkins discovered the 'sew-in' method. Today, the wig and weave industry is huge, with women of all backgrounds partaking in this hair culture.

SHAVED

Hair can be shaved with clippers to obtain a short cut across the whole head.

Some Black women decide to shave their head as a key step in transitioning from relaxed to curly hair. This gets rid of any damaged and relaxed hair, allowing the hair to start afresh and grow back totally natural. This is known as the 'big chop' and is a key moment in some naturalistas' hair journeys.

Many Black women enjoy shorter hair because it's less maintenance than longer hair, and others like that they are rejecting mainstream standards of beauty that promote long, straight hair. No matter how short one's hair is, it should still be cleansed and moisturised regularly in order to stay healthy.

LAYING YOUR EDGES

Edges, also known as baby hairs, are small, short hairs found around the hairline. Hair gels are used to style the edges and hold them into place. The practice of 'laying your edges' has long been a feature of Black hair styling, originating in the 1900s.[10] The desire to have slicked down edges came from attempts to reflect European ideals on Black hair.[11] By the 1920s, the practice became standard amongst Black women who would use products to flatten and reshape the hair on their hairline.[12] Today, laying your edges remains a hair styling staple amongst Black women with non-Black women also adopting the style.

As common as it is, 'laying your edges' often can cause dryness, flakiness and breakage. It's important to wet hair that has been hardened by gel so that it softens and is less brittle before being brushed, to minimise breakage.

9

THE CURLS AND COILS
OF SOCIAL MEDIA

Without the internet, it's unlikely that the contemporary natural hair movement would have occurred in the way it did. The modern iteration of the natural hair movement started in the 2000s and peaked around the years of 2008 and 2009. It began in the USA with the boom of social media. Black women began sharing information, images and videos pertaining to their natural hair journeys and hair care routines. Sites like Google, YouTube and later, Instagram and TikTok opened up a world of possibilities for Black women and their hair care. Due to the popularity of relaxers and straighteners, many Black women weren't too familiar with their natural coils and how to manage them when transitioning from relaxed hair. The internet was an effective way to fill in that knowledge gap.

When asked about what factors positively influenced Black women's relationship with their hair, 77% of the participants of my survey selected social media.

Social media has transformed the way Black women view their hair journeys. What was once a very personal and private relationship has become a communal experience shared with multiple people all over the world through various platforms. A thesis by Jené M Shepherd found that women with Afro-textured hair view social media platforms as a safe space—a place where they can access emotional support whilst navigating their hair journeys and embracing their identities.[1]

Many Black women have reported that they felt inspired to transition back to natural hair due to seeing other Black women on social media do so. Before the social media boom, it was difficult for Black women to access accurate and digestible information on hair care outside of one's direct social circle. In this sense, the internet created a larger and more expansive Black hair network also known as 'naturalistas' or 'curlies'.

ANECDOTES FROM THE 'BLACK WOMEN AND THEIR HAIR' SURVEY

'The natural hair movement among Black YouTubers, seeing the breath of natural hairstyles and watching someone on the journey of loving their natural hair was inspiring.'

'Seeing Black women on social media (Instagram, YouTube) showcase their hair and what they do with it really helped to integrate the idea that my hair can and should be worn however I want. I can and should be indulgent with what I use on it and love the process of caring for it. These women have helped to normalise Black hair in the cosmetic world. I feel like hair is very intimate and sacred for Black women because, like many people, we want it to be beautiful, to feel beautiful. But there are very little spaces for us to express it. As usual, Black women created these spaces themselves online and it helped me to feel good about my own hair.'

'My relationship with my curls has been a long one and with regards to social media, it's incredible to see people

celebrating their natural hair. I definitely have felt more
comfortable and part of a community, having come
from a place where my hair was very different from
everyone else's.'

As a millennial, the internet has similarly played a major
role in my hair care. Up until recently, I never knew how to
canerow my hair (yes, that's right, some Black women do not
know how to canerow!). My mum and my sisters styled my
hair for me up until I left home for university, so I never felt
the need to learn. Once I was at university, I either left my hair
out or I used hair straighteners. However, after graduating, it
suddenly dawned on me that 1) not being able to canerow my
hair was preventing me from trying out the cool hair styles I
saw on social media, and 2) if I were to have a child in future,
I wouldn't be able to canerow their hair or teach them how to
do it themselves.

Throughout history, Black hairstyling techniques have
been passed down from generation to generation, and I did
not want that to stop at me. So, did I wallow in my inability
to be a supreme canerower? Of course not! I did what any
logical woman would do and watched countless tutorials on
YouTube until I was able to canerow my own hair—a long and
exhausting process, but worth it in the end!

VLOGGING AND INFLUENCING

Much of the information that Black women are able to access
on natural hair care came via what is now known as the vlogger
and the social media influencer.

VLOGGER: An individual who creates personal videos that
feature themselves, their life or their expertise as the main

subject, usually uploading video content onto YouTube or similar social media platforms.

SOCIAL MEDIA INFLUENCER: Someone who has established credibility on an online space usually pertaining to a particular industry or skill set, causing them to gain a large audience and the ability to influence their followers and fans.

Vloggers and social media influencers in the natural hair space use their platforms to educate their followers through sharing hair care routines, reviewing hair products, posting tutorials for hairstyles and much more. YouTube videos of vloggers documenting their natural hair journeys can be found with hundreds of thousands of views, and in some cases, millions. Similarly, Instagram reviews of hair products rack up impressive engagement levels. More recently, newer social media applications like TikTok have also entered the natural hair content game with countless tutorials uploaded to the app each day.

Due to the success of the online Black hair space, vlogging and influencing has become a viable and lucrative career option for some. Hair brands, both big and small, have noticed this and begun infiltrating this space, partnering with vloggers and influencers to promote and sell their products.

The contemporary natural hair movement did not occur in a vacuum. It coincided with several movements that all found a home online and rapidly grew. These movements included the body positivity movement, which promotes the acceptance and normalisation of diverse body types,[2] the health and wellness movement which aims to promote the importance and maintenance of our physical and mental health, and the sustainability movement, which pushes people to assess how their lifestyles impact the environment, promoting the use of environmentally-friendly products. The growth of these movements in the 2000s promoted constructive ideals that encouraged us to live better and be better to others.

The natural hair hair movement of the 2000s, whilst widely seen as positive, is not without criticism. Ironically, one critique of the movement is that it failed and continues to fail to be truly inclusive. Now, I think it is important to state that this iteration of the natural hair movement is perhaps the most impactful to date with Black women becoming more privy to the science and health of their hair in a way that we have not seen before, however, even with all the positives, it still falls victim to colourism and texturism.

'The natural movement has been co-opted by mixed heritage women with soft curls already.'
—Survey Participant.

The natural hair movement is intended to represent all Black women and the diversity of all Black hair types. However, the movement has been accused of making women with looser, Type 3 hair the face of the movement, overlooking Black women with coily Type 4 hair. The criticism follows a similar pattern that has appeared in the body positivity movement, which it has been accused of idolising curvy, toned bodies with small waists rather than all body types.

In the case of the natural hair movement, the centering of Type 3 hair excludes the experience and importance of Type 4 hair, which is arguably the hair type that needs the movement most.

Shepherd's 2018 thesis explored texturism within the natural hair community, specifically on social media. Shepherd analysed the 75 best- and worst-performing social media posts of three brands specifically catering to Afro-textured hair and assessed the comments on each post and what the sentiments were around them.[3]

When these brands posted content that advertised their products, they generally used lighter-skinned models. These adverts are there to promote the product and show how beautiful people's hair can look when using it. By using models of lighter skin tones, and therefore most likely looser curls, this sends out the message that Type 3 curls are the aspiration. The comments from users reflected this, with many displaying envy of the model's curls.

'Almost all of the models featured in posts which left commenters lusting after their curls in the comments section had Type 3, curly hair. Given the findings that a disproportionate amount of the models featured in these images feature curly hair, commenters are praising and idealizing this hair type.'[4]

It's difficult to determine whether commenters feel this way because the brands are posting a disproportionate amount of images with Type 3 hair, or whether the brands are posting these images more frequently than other hair types because they know that this drives greater engagement. Unfortunately, the cycle of texturism continues, and this sends a message that only a certain type of natural hair is worthy of being platformed.

Much of the criticism and frustration surrounding the natural hair movement are voiced by Black women online. In this sense the internet, yet again, provides a ground for Black women to discuss and share their opinions of a movement and how it can be improved. On Twitter, there have been many viral tweets made by Black women stating the sidelining of

Type 4 hair within the natural hair movement.

One of my survey participants described the impact that the centering of Type 3 hair had on her.

'My further frustration is that I have been natural
for 6 years and my hair only reaches my shoulders. I
expected my hair to stretch down to the bottom of my
back because that's all I see on social media […] When
my hair was relaxed, I was never confident because it
would never go past my chin so I thought, since I'm
natural it should be healthy and long. But that didn't
happen, it's longer than the relaxed hair but still not
long enough. I still catch myself longing for Type 3
hair […] I feel like I was sold this dream by the natural
hair community that my hair should be down to my tail
bone within 4 years. It's been 6 years and my hair just
touches my shoulders.'

The lack of representation of Type 4 hair, at times, does appear to be a deliberate exclusion of Black women with the kinkiest hair, who are usually those with darker skin. This serves as a reminder of how deep-rooted the influence of racism within the world of Black hair is, even within movements that appear to push against such views.

When we think of well-known 'naturalistas', we rarely think of an individual with Type 4 hair. If the natural hair industry is anything to go by, Type 4 hair is only accepted and enjoyed when it imitates the textures of other hair types. The image of long, loose and bouncy curls is the image of natural hair that has been pushed and promoted. This is not to say that Type 3 hair does not deserve representation and acceptance because it certainly does. However, out of all the hair textures that Black women have, Type 4 hair is the most negatively viewed and stereotyped. Social media representation of naturalistas and imagery pertaining to natural hair clearly reflects this texturism, with Type 3 hair attaining exposure that Type 4 hair does not.

Given that the rhetoric around Type 4 hair, even within the natural movement, reinforces ideals about its untamable and deviant behaviour, the natural hair movement has more work to do before it can claim to be truly inclusive. The language surrounding 4C hair in particular focuses on how challenging it can be to handle, the hair's fragility and how prone it is to breakage. Whilst some of these statements are true, there seems to be a far stronger focus on these features in comparison to other Black hair types.

So, can the sidelining of kinky hair within the natural hair movement change? And if so, how?

An increase in the amount of Type 4 hair representation in adverts, films, music videos, social media would assist in normalising Type 4 hair. Seeing Type 4 hair is a rarity, so much so that when it does occur, it is a memorable cultural moment; we all remember our surprise when we watched Annalise Keating (played by Viola Davis) remove her wig to reveal her Type 4 natural hair in hit show *How To Get Away With Murder*. The surprise was rooted in the fact that this is an image that we very rarely see in popular culture and mainstream media.

The natural hair movement also needs to refrain from centring a specific type of curly hair that is not shared by all Black women. Instead, the health of the hair should be the focus. Attempting to imitate curls purely for aesthetic reasons is not what true inclusivity of all hair types looks like.

Kinky, coily, natural Black hair deserves to be recognised and for the natural hair movement to achieve its intended purpose, it is essential that this is the case.

INTERVIEW WITH HAIR INFLUENCER BEULAH DAVINA

Someone who has been dedicated to highlighting kinky, coily Black hair is Black British natural hair influencer Beulah Davina. For a long time, Black Brits would look to the Black community in the US for advice and guidance on all things Black hair and products. Today, with the growth and popularity of the Black British hair industry, the visibility of Black British naturalistas has also increased. I spoke to Beulah Davina who is the founder of The Creamy Crack Rehab, an Instagram page dedicated to all things natural hair. Davina created the page in 2015 when she decided to embark on her natural hair journey.

ZKS: How did you build your social media platform and what do you hope to achieve through it? Was it always a goal of yours to have a platform like The Creamy Crack Rehab?

BD: I built my social media platform initially for myself. I stopped relaxing my hair and had no idea how to look after my natural texture, so I created a platform for me to curate images and information to help me through the process. I made the blog public so that others could use it if they needed to, but I had no idea it would become what it is now. Seven years on, I'm pretty clued up on all things hair so now I'm just hoping my content inspires, educates and entertains.

ZKS: What challenges have you faced being a Black natural hair influencer on social media? What have some of the highlights been?

BD: In the natural hair industry, looser curls and lighter skin are favoured so as a dark-skinned, kinky-haired influencer I've definitely found that I haven't been granted the same opportunities or access as others who fit the desired aesthetic. I've also found at times that I've been the token dark skin influencer in campaigns, which is frustrating.

The highlights are the free products (natural hair products can be pricey lol) and the community that has been built online and offline. I've made some amazing friends because of my job.

ZKS: How has your engagement changed over the years? Are you finding that there is certain content that your followers engage with more than others?

BD: The number one thing people come to my platform for is hair content, but over the past few years I've also been known for the memes and illustrations I create. Some of the illustrations I created this year have the highest engagement of all the content I've created and some of them have nothing to do with hair and actually tackle political issues. Twenty twenty has been one of the most politically turbulent years of my adulthood so this doesn't surprise me.

ZKS: What are your thoughts of the positive and/or negative effects social media has on the natural hair movement or people's relationships with their hair?

BD: Social media tends to encourage comparison and I think comparing your hair to anyone else's can be dangerous. From growth rate, to length and texture, you'll always find someone with hair that you desire more than your own so self-love and acceptance is a must.

A positive effect of social media is the community. The natural hair journey isn't easy for everyone and social media provides resources, information, tools and friendships that make the journey easier.

Whilst the internet and social media provided a fruitful environment for Black hair care, the internet is not always a place of positivity for Black women.

Back when I was 19 years old, around the time the natural hair movement was taking its reign on social media, I was mindlessly tweeting to my (very small number of) followers about a new song that I did not like. Within minutes, a complete stranger who ran a fan account for the artist tweeted me, telling me that I needed to relax my hair because my Afro looked like I had been electrocuted.

If you are unfamiliar with Twitter, specifically Black Twitter at that time, such a response may seem shocking and unwarranted. However, whilst the movements (natural hair; body positivity; health and wellness) were gradually seeping into the online ether, this was also a time where the expression of colourism on social media was commonplace. This was a time where it was not surprising for young Black people to see tweets and posts about the unattractiveness of 'nappy' natural hair, disgust at Black women who wore weaves and the oddly strong disdain for Black women wearing braids.

The social media timelines of young Black people were littered with YouTube clips of young men from the UK being stopped in the street and asked what their type or preference was when it came to women—they almost always responded with 'mixed-race girls' or a 'lightie'. As a dark-skinned Black girl with Afro hair, being on social media during that time was rough. You were not only made to feel invisible at times, but your entire being was made to feel unwanted and undesirable. Black women, their hair and their skin tone were the butt of all the jokes.

At times, it is hard to imagine that it is the same social media apps that helped carve out a community for Black women to exchange and learn about their hair, Blackness and identity in later years, were also a place where Black girls and women were (and still are) vilified and cyber-abused.

GEORGE FLOYD & COVID-19

The murder of George Floyd in 2020 led to world wide protests and a resurgence in the Black Lives Matter movement. The public outrage and pain spilled over into industries and institutions. Suddenly, brands were being held to account in a way that we had never seen before and challenged on what they were doing for the Black community.

In terms of Black hair care, we started seeing hair companies publicly showing their support for the Black Lives Matter movement through effective social media campaigns, advertising and donations to Black charities and organisations. At the start of 2021, Pantene launched a campaign called 'My Hair Won't Be Silenced' featuring Black British women sharing their experiences of hair discrimination. The campaign was a collaboration with Project Embrace, which aims to increase positive media representation of Afro-textured hair, and Black Minds Matter, a charity which provides mental health services to Black people. Pantene conducted a study that revealed 93% of Black people in the UK experience hair discrimintation. This campaign was also associated with Pantene's new Afro hair care range, the Pantene Gold Series, which was created by Black scientists.

Hair and beauty companies began speaking up about and supporting Black lives. Being that Black customers, specifically Black women, have largely been ignored by the industry, the sudden attention was quite a surprise for many. This push to focus on Black lives and customers also led to the spotlight being placed on Black-owned businesses. The need to support Black businesses was seen as a useful and practical way of showing solidarity with the Black community, with allies and Black consumers making a concerted effort to buy from Black-owned businesses. This shift would lead to campaigns such as Black Pound Day, where on the first Saturday of every month, consumers are asked to exclusively shop with Black-owned businesses.

Black-owned hair and beauty brands were able to galvanise their social media and internet output to effectively capitalize on the sudden demand for Black-owned products.

When the COVID lockdown led to the closure of places of businesses, the hair salon and the hair shop industry ceased. Black women were now staying at home, having to manage their hair without the assistance they were perhaps accustomed too. For some hair specialists and businesses, this provided an opportunity to educate and help Black women. Experts, like trichologist Ebuni Adijuah, sought to educate Black women by conducting online hair tutorials as well as group video sessions for Black women who wanted to do their hair together and have their hair questions answered. Black women also moved towards adopting a more DIY approach when it came to their hair care, creating homemade products and experimenting with ingredients.

So when it comes to the importance of social media and the internet in relation to natural Black hair care, it is a major pillar. It has given Black women like myself a place to see that we are not alone in our hair journeys and has dramatically widened our knowledge pool. Simultaneously, social media and the internet have also been a space where many Black women of my generation have seen or been subject to texturism and misogynoir. Yes, it's a double-edged sword, but its prominence and positive impact cannot be ignored.

Would there be this latest iteration of the natural hair movement without social media and the internet? I am not sure there would be.

CONCLUSION

UNTANGLING OUR FUTURE

We have almost reached the end of our time together. The exploration of Black women and their natural hair can, at times, bring more questions with it than answers. But sometimes, these questions are just as important. One particularly important one is *what is the future of Black women and their Afro hair?*

Technology has played a huge role in how Black women care for and learn about their hair. From YouTube hair vloggers to Instagram naturalistas, the centrality of technology in the world of Black hair gets stronger year on year.

Afrocks is a Black-British-owned online platform that works to connect clients with mobile Afro hairdressers. When I spoke to Stella Lucien and Simone Williamson from Afrocks, they explained that the founder of the company created the company after being, 'frustrated about the time it took for him to find a good stylist.' Afrocks gives clients a quick and easy way to book and pay for their appointments online, whilst providing a formal booking system for mobile hairstylists. Customers are able to discover new high-quality hairstylists through the platform. Lucien and Williamson tell me, 'We have competency-based interviews with the mobile hairstylists, background check them and check their experience as well as their portfolio. We want to provide a good service to clients so we make sure hairstylists understand the level of service we expect.'

Another key focus is providing guidance to the mobile hairstylists to help them with the running of their business. 'A lot of hairstylists learn in very informal settings. So it's hard to make that transition into business when it's something that you've been doing as a hobby since you were young and you probably did it for free. With Afrocks, we wanted to streamline the professionalism process.'

Carra is a new online platform that launched during the COVID-19 pandemic, to provide customers with a highly tailored hair care service. The platform, founded by Winnie Awa, asks users a series of questions relating to their hair journey and uses this to provide access to product recommendations, personalised hair care routines and one-on-one consultations with hair coaches. In my interview with Winnie, she explained that, 'we hear the same things often: "how do I care for my hair?", "how do I do this without spending hours on YouTube?", "how do I know the best products and ingredients for my hair?" We are re-envisioning today's noisy and overwhelming textured hair experience to build a truly borderless personalisation platform targeting multicultural women all across the globe.'

In short, technology has the power to make the Black hair styling experience more streamlined, connected and simple for customers as well as for those providing hair care services.

The increase in Black hair innovators has led non-Black organisations to similarly create spaces for Black hair. In August 2021, we saw online platform Pinterest launch a feature called 'hair pattern', allowing users of the site to search and filter content by a specific hair texture and type.[1] With online algorithms defaulting to a narrow selection of hair types, the 'hair pattern' tool puts the power back into the hands of the user, allowing them to find the content that truly matters and relates to them. Going forward, the accessibility and discover-ability of content regarding Black hair care will continue to improve. As the industry learns more about Black hair, moves like Pinterest's will only increase.

The natural hair care product market is expected to grow at an annual rate of 4.7% internationally, reaching the value of $12.7 billion by the year 2027.[2] Today, we are seeing more Black-owned brands become serious players in the hair care industry, and it will be interesting to observe whether they will dominate the market by increased sales and greater involve-ment in every step of the supply chain. This could be achieved by Black people pursuing careers not only as retailers, but as manufacturers and distributors too. Black-owned hair compa-nies adopting a collaborative strategy will enable them to gain greater purchasing power as a collective, offering more com-petitive prices to their customers and thus generating more profit.

In terms of this present-day natural hair movement, I believe that it will continue to go forth and have a lasting impact on Black women and their hair care. The continued focus on hair health over hair type or hair length has the potential to truly empower Black women and support them on their hair journeys like never before. My hope is that the current natural hair movement becomes even more inclusive, celebrating all curly and coily hair textures, particularly 4C hair.

There is a lot of noise surrounding Black women's natural hair, much of which is not rooted in facts. It is therefore imper-ative that the natural hair movement evolves into becoming less complex and teaching Black women about the science of their hair, what products they should not use and what ingre-dients are healthy. The current natural hair movement has gotten better in these areas, but we are still sold a plethora of products promising to give us curl definition like never before or we are told that if we follow a 'simple' ELEVEN-step routine, our hair will grow at a faster rate. What is needed is for Black women to understand their hair. This takes time, and is often learnt through both experimentation and research. Once we begin to focus solely on what our hair needs to stay healthy, Afro hair care should become simpler.

The desired image of Black women's hair is still entrenched in the idea of aesthetic 'perfection'. Not a single hair should be out of place. This prevents us from fully accepting the diversity of natural Afro hair. Laying our edges is fun and stylish but it is OK if some baby hairs aren't fully gelled into place or if the edges aren't laid at all! Immaculate curls are great but so is frizz. Much of the pressure of perfection within the world of Black women and their hair has deeply problematic roots, as we have explored within this book. The de-perfection of Black hair is a development that will allow us to not only normalise the diversity of our hair, but also focus on the health of our hair rather than how it appears.

The modern natural hair movement exploded in the way that it did due to the rapid dissemination of information and content through social media. We have huge online Black hair communities providing support and guidance to millions of young women. Despite society becoming increasingly digital, I believe physical spaces could still play an important role in the future, and bring these online communities to life in person. Imagine if there was a place where you could buy all your hair products, get your hair done, learn new styling techniques or just get some general hair care guidance all in one? Imagine if there was a place for young Black girls to learn to embrace and celebrate their hair and be exposed to Black women of all hair types, textures and styles? Imagine if that same place held fun support groups for those of us who STILL can't canerow! There's an opportunity to reimagine and recreate the hair salon into a place that caters to the ever-evolving needs of Black hair.

The pandemic and the resurgence of the Black Lives Matter movement due to the tragic killing of George Floyd resulted in many changes in the future of Black hair care. Some were more permanent than others. Consumer behaviour has shifted to purchases being made almost exclusively through digital platforms, with many high-street shops closing down due to lack of sales. At the same time, there has been an increase in support for Black-owned businesses. Only time will tell us whether this support will translate into real, tangible change for these businesses. Effective Black British marketplaces such as HairPopp and Jamii provide platforms for consumers to discover Black-owned brands. Black-owned hair care subscription service Treasure Tress similarly thrived during the pandemic.

There have also been other developments such as consumers seeking more sustainable, healthier hair products. It is of course hard to predict what new trends will crop up or what new information we will have access to in the future. But as we have seen, when it comes to Black hair, when we know better, we seem to do better, and the more we'll see positive change come about.

The internet will continue to permit global conversations about Black hair care. We, of course, cannot prognosticate what new social media app will be the next big thing, but have enough evidence to see that whatever it is, the Black hair community will use it to disseminate information, just as they did with YouTube, Instagram, Twitter and, more recently, Clubhouse and TikTok.

What are my hopes for the future of Black women and their hair? That we can create a world where the trauma of having natural hair no longer exists. That we can live in a world where Black girls and women can exist without having to go through what Ruby Williams went through. I believe that this will only become possible once legislation such as the CROWN Act has been been passed in more US states, and when the UK decides to implement a similar law to protect Black people from hair discrimination. In the meantime, more schools and companies in the UK need to review hair and uniform policies that may be discriminatory, and sign up to the Halo Code to prove their commitment to fighting for this cause.

I hope for a Black hair future that gives space and support to those of us who experience the height of racism, texturism and colourism. We should see more dark-skinned women and girls with Type 4C hair brandished on campaigns, adverts and products. Simply put, we must decolonise the natural hair industry.

The language we use to speak about Afro hair needs to change. We must refrain from speaking about our hair as a nuisance, as problematic, as something unworthy of being seen and celebrated. This is done through many means, but specifically education. Learning about the history of our hair and why so many of us have been conditioned to deem it undesirable, gives us the context and knowledge to understand why such conditioning is wrong and harmful.

Finally, I hope we can one day live in a world where natural Black hair in all its diversity is celebrated and seen as beautiful—because it is!

ENDNOTES

PREFACE

1   Ejindu, Thandi. "Afro Hair... Don't Care!" *Huffington Post*, 18 February 2016

CHAPTER 2

1   Byrd, Ayana D., and Lori L. Tharps. *Hair Story: Untangling the Roots of Black Hair in America*. St. Martin's Griffin, 2001

2   Ibid.

3   Bohela, Tulanana. "Tanzania's Maasai: From warriors to hairdressers." *BBC*, 23 June 2015

4   Dabiri, Emma. *Don't Touch My Hair*, Penguin Books, 2019, p. 33.

5   Byrd, Ayana D., and Lori L. Tharps. *Hair Story: Untangling the Roots of Black Hair: Untangling the Roots of Black Hair in America*, St Martin's Press, 2002, p. 8-10.

6   Ibid.

7   Carney, Judith A. "'With Grains in Her Hair': Rice in Colonial Brazil." *Slavery and Abolition*, vol. 25, no. 1, 2004

8   Dabiri, Emma. *Don't Touch My Hair*, Penguin Books, 2019, p. 229

9   Brown, DeNeen. *Afro-Colombian women braid messages of freedom in hairstyles*. The Washington Post, 2011

10   Dabiri, Emma. *Don't Touch My Hair*, Penguin Books, 2019, p. 117

11   Abolition of the transatlantic slave trade." *National Museums Liverpool*, Liverpool Museums, https://www.

liverpoolmuseums.org.uk/history-of-slavery/abolition.

12   Cumming, Valerie, et al. *The Dictionary of Fashion History*, Bloomsbury Publishing, 2017, p. 128.

13   Gates, Jr., Henry Louis. "Madam Walker, the First Black American Woman to Be a Self-Made Millionaire." *pbs. org*, PBS, 2004

14   "Garrett Morgan Biography." *Biography.com*, A&E Television Networks, 2014

15   Dabiri, Emma. *Don't Touch My Hair*, Penguin Books, 2019, p. 107-108.

16   Byrd, Ayana D., and Lori L. Tharps. *Hair Story: Untangling the Roots of Black Hair: Untangling the Roots of Black Hair in America*, St Martin's Press, 2002, p. 31,35.

17   Dyke, Dryden and Wade entrepreneurs." *Black Plaque Project.*

18   Ibid.

19   Sherrow, Victoria. "Johnson Products." *Encyclopedia of Hair: A Cultural History*, Greenwood Press, 2006, p. 229.

20   Kusmer, Kenneth L., and Joe W. Trotter. "Black Dollar Power." *African American Urban History since World War II (Historical Studies of Urban America)*, University of Chicago Press, 2009, p. 402.

21   Byrd, Ayana D., and Lori L. Tharps. *Hair Story: Untangling the Roots of Black Hair: Untangling the Roots of Black Hair in America*. St Martin's Press, 2002.

22   Ibid.

23   Wade, Tony. *How They Made a Million: The Dyke and Dryden Story*, Hansib Publications, 2001, p. 57

24   Tharps, Lori L. *Hair Story: Untangling the Roots of Black Hair in America*, St Martin's Press, 2002, p. 118.

CHAPTER 3

1   Norwood, Kimberly Jade. ""If You Is White, You's Alright..." Stories About Colorism in America." *Washington University Global Studies Law Review*, vol. 14, no. 4, 2015

2   Seakamela, Shasha. "BLACK HAIR—BRIDGING A 'CODE OF CONDUCT.'" *Fair Planet*, 20 September 2016

3   Ibid.

4   Pearn Kandola. "Racism at Work Survey Results." *Pearn Kandola*, March 2018.

5   Rosette, Ashleigh Shelby, and Christy Zhou Koval. "The Natural Hair Bias in Job Recruitment." *Social Psychological and Personality Science*, vol. 12, 2020

6   McCluney, Courtney L., et al. "The Costs of Code-Switching." *Harvard Business Review*, 15 November 2019

7   BBC News. "Fulham schoolboy dreadlock ban overturned." *BBC*, 12 September 2018,

8   Gutierrez-Morfin, Noel. "U.S. Court Rules Dreadlock Ban During Hiring Process Is Legal." *NBC News*, 21 September 2016

CHAPTER 4

1   DeAngelis, Tori. "Unmasking 'racial micro aggressions'. Monitor on Psychology, 40(2).

2   Solorzano, Daniel, et al. "Critical Race Theory, Racial Microaggressions, and Campus Racial Climate: The Experiences of African American College Students." *The Journal of Negro Education*, vol. 69, no. 1/2, 2000, pp. 60-73.

3   Pantene. "Help end Afro hair discrimination." *https://www.pantene.co.uk/*, 2021

4   The University of Edinburgh. "Effects of Microaggressions." *The University of Edinburgh*

5   Ibid.

6   Underwood, Khalea. "Hey, Kim Kardashian: These Are Not "Bo Derek Braids."" *Refinery29*, 29 January 2018

7   Ibid.

8   Kalter, Suzy. "In An Odd Twist, from 10, the Beauty Biz Finds the Cornrow Is Oh, So Green." *People Magazine*, 11 February 1980

9   YouTube. "Paul Mooney: Everyone Wants To Be A N*gga." *YouTube*, 16 June 2016

10   Fonrouge, Gabrielle. "The story of Rachel Dolezal gets even more bizarre." *The New York Post*

11   Grinberg, Emanuella. "Perm or weave? Rachel Dolezal puts hair questions to rest." *CNN*

CHAPTER 5

1   Bourne, Stephen. "Obituary: Pauline Henriques." *The Independent*, 21 November 1998

2   Ibid.

3   BBC. "PROGRAMME INDEX." *BBC Television*, 1946

4   Bourne, Stephen. "Obituary: Pauline Henriques." *The Independent*, 21 November 1998

5   Ibid.

6   Jolaoso, Simi. "Barbara Blake Hannah: The first black female reporter on British TV." *BBC News*, 23 October 2020

7   Jones, Ellen E. "Barbara Blake-Hannah: how Britain's first black female TV reporter was forced off our screens." *The Guardian*, 7 January 2021

8   Bruno, Natasha. "Texture Talk: 3 Fashion Week Pros on the Importance of Industry-Wide Textured Hair Education." *Fashion Magazine*, Fashion Magazine, 2021

9   March, Bridget. "Jourdan Dunn reveals why she has

to wear wigs." *Cosmopolitan*, 26 March 2016

10   Ibid.

11   *Grazia* Magazine. "Leomie Anderson: 'As A Black Model You Can't Just Be And Exist.'" *Grazia*, 19 June 2020

12   Ibid.

13   Ibid.

14   Andrews, Jessica. "Model Olivia Anakwe Calls Out Hairstylists Who Can't Do Black Hair at Fashion Shows." *Teen Vogue*, 8 March 2019

15   Ibid.

16   Ibid.

17   Andrews, Jessica. "Naomi Campbell Talks About The Discrimination Black Models Face at Fashion Week." *Teen Vogue*, 14 March 2016.

18   Hughes, Sali. "Alek Wek: 'You don't have to go with the crowd.'" *The Guardian*, 28 March 2014

19   BBC Sounds—100 Women. "Interview: Alek Wek—Model." *BBC*, 2015

20   Elan, Priya. "Survey finds that 78% of models in fashion adverts are white." *The Guardian*, 10 May 2016

21   Krupnick, Ellie. "This White Model Is Rocking an Afro in Allure Magazine, and People Are Upset." *MIC*, 3 August 2015

22   Allen, Maya. "This White Model Is Getting Props for the Way She Apologized for Her Blackhair Cover." *Cosmopolitan Magazine*, 28 November 2016

23   Ibid.

24   Petter, Olivia. "Vogue apologises after Kendall Jenner photoshoot is criticised for 'cultural appropriation.'" *The Independent*, 24 October 2018

25   Ibid

26   Russo, Gianluca. "8 Times Fashion Designers Have Appropriated Black Hairstyles at Fashion Week." *Teen Vogue*

27   *The Voice*. "The Untold Story Of Britain's First Black Female Superstar." *The Voice*, 30 March 2017

28   Ibid.

29   Hebblethwaite, Phil. "Black and British: iconic images of our music stars from the BBC archive." *BBC*, 11 November 2016

30   TIGG, FNR. "Mathew Knowles Thinks Beyonce's Lighter Skin Helped Her Career." *Complex*, 19 June 2019

31   Buxton, Ryan. "Mel B Explains Where The Nickname Scary Spice Came From." *Huffington Post*, 15 September 2015

32   Storey, Katie. "Mel B gets real honest about her experience of racism and recalls standing her ground over her 'identity' in the Spice Girls." *Metro*, 7 June 2020

33   Ibid.

34   Beaumont-Thomas, Ben. "Alexandra Burke says music industry told her to bleach her skin." *The Guardian*, 20 June 2020

35   Ibid.

36   BBC Newsround. "Jamelia: I wanted to look like my idols." *BBC*, 14 September 2018

37   Ibid.

38   Ibid.

39   Mussen, Madeline. "The heart-wrenching reason why presenter Rochelle Humes decided to change her hair." *My London*, 9 April 2021

40   "Rochelle Humes Reveals How Her Daughter Inspired Her New Book." *This Morning*, created by ITV, 7 February 2019

CHAPTER 6

1   Ejindu, Thandi. "Afro Hair... Don't Care!" *Huffington Post*, 18 February 2016

2   Mintel Press Office. "Naturally confident: More than half of Black women say their hair makes them feel beautiful." *Mintel*, 9 October 2018

3   Ejindu, Thandi. "Afro Hair... Don't Care!" *Huffington Post*, 18 February 2016

4   Mamona, Sheilla. "This is why black women unfairly spend so much money on their hair." *Glamour*, 15 October 2020

5   Institute of Practitioners in Advertising. "2012 Multicultural Britain." *IPA*, 2012

6   Bryd, Ayana D., and Lori L. Tharps. *Hair Story: Untangling the Roots of Black Hair in America*, St. Martin's Griffin, 2001, pp. 83-84.

7   Ibid.

8   Genzlinger, Neil. "Joan Johnson, Whose Company Broke a Racial Barrier, Dies at 89." *The New York Times*, 10 September 2019

9   Reuters Staff. "UPDATE 1-P&G sells Johnson Products hair care unit." *Reuters*, 31 March 2009

10   "How to remake your company like Johnson Products." *Black Enterprise*, 19 July 2010

11   American Health and Beauty Aids Institute. "About ABHAI." *AHBAI*, 2021

12   Ibid

13   Farhi, Paul. "HAIR CARE BATTLE LINES DRAWN IN BLACK, WHITE." *The Washington Post*, 27 December 1993

14   Ibid

15   Ibid

16   Ibid

17   Sylbourne Sydial TV Show. "Tony Wade of Dyke & Dryden—one of Britain's "first Black Millionaires"—PART 1." *YouTube*, 25 August 2015

18   Byrd, Ayana D., and Lori L. Tharps. *Hair Story:*

Untangling the Roots of Black Hair in America. St. Martin's Griffin, 2001

19   The Federation of Small Businesses (FSB). "Unlocking opportunity: The value of ethnic minority firms to UK economic activity and enterprise." 2020, p. 19. FSB

20   Mintel Press Office. "Naturally confident: More than half of Black women say their hair makes them feel beautiful." *Mintel,* 9 October 2018

21   Ibid.

CHAPTER 7

1   Britannica, The Editors of Encyclopaedia. "pH". Encyclopedia Britannica, 3 Jun. 2020

2   Food and Drug Administration. "Cosmetics Labeling Guide." *U.S. Food and Drug Administration*

3   Centers for Disease Control and Prevention. "Phthalates Factsheet." *Centers for Disease Control and Prevention*

4   National Institutes of Health. "Permanent hair dye and straighteners may increase breast cancer risk." *National Institutes of Health,* 4 December 2019

CHAPTER 8

1   Smith, Kim. "STRANDS OF THE SIXTIES A Cultural Analysis of the Design and Consumption Of the New London West End Hair Salons c. 1954-1975." 2014, p. 218

2   Ibid.

3   Brinkhurst-Cuff, Charlie. "Should We Be Encouraging White Hairdressers To Learn How To Do Black Hair?" Refinery29, 21 June 2017

4   Bencosme, Yamilex. "Beauty is Pain: Black Women's Identity and Their Struggle with Embracing Their Natural

Hair." *Perspectives*, vol. Vol. 9 , Article 1, 2017

5   Ring, Kyle. "Twisted Locks of Hair: The Complicated History of Dreadlocks." Esquire, 26 October 2020

6   Ibid.

7   Ibid.

8   Crowhurst, Anna-Marie. "Remembering Christina Jenkins, the woman who invented the weave." *Stylist Magazine*, November 2018

9   Ibid.

10   Uhai Hair. "Baby Hairs: The History of Edges & Edge Control." *Medium*, 11 August 2020.

11   Ibid.

12   "'Stiff where?' It's time to talk about our damaging addiction to laid edges." *Gal-dem*, 18 February 2021

CHAPTER 9

1   Shepherd, Jené M. "Don't touch my crown: Texturism as an extension of colorism in the natural hair community." 2018

2   Lazuka, Rebecca F., et al. "Are We There Yet? Progress in Depicting Diverse Images of Beauty in Instagram's Body Positivity Movement." *Science Direct*, vol. 34, 2020, pp. 85-93. *Science Direct*,

3   Shepherd, Jené M. "Don't touch my crown: Texturism as an extension of colorism in the natural hair community." 2018

4   Ibid.

CONCLUSION

1   DALL'ASEN, NICOLA. "Pinterest's New Feature Lets You Filter Hair Searches by Texture or Type." *Allure*, 18

August 2021

2   Grand View Research. "Natural Hair Care Product Market Size, Share & Trends Analysis Report By End Use (Men, Women),." *Grand View Research*, 2020

ACKNOWLEDGEMENTS

Firstly, I would like to thank Mags, Magdalene Abraha, the mother of *A Quick Ting On* whom I feel lucky to call my friend. Wow, what a journey it's been! Thank you for inviting me to be part of this revolutionary series and providing me with support at every step of the way. Never in a million years would I have considered publishing a book, and I can't thank you enough for seeing the potential in me.

To my beautiful mum, who raised me to become the woman I am today. Thank you for showering me with love and teaching me that I can achieve anything that I want to in life. Nakupenda.

My amazing big sisters, my first ever friends, Zahra and Bishara. Where do I begin? You both inspired me to be bold, confident and comfortable in my own skin. Thank you for being such great role models and for always having my back... and my scalp. From parting my hair and laying my edges, to straightening my hair after I would beg you to do it, I appreciate the guidance you have both given me as I navigated my hair journey over the years. You don't know how much you have both positively influenced me.

Shout out to my best friends (you know who you are) for your constant encouragement, for allowing me to pick your brains when I had a mind blank or wanted to explore ideas for the book, and for helping me to proofread sections and transcribe interviews. I'm so grateful for the virtual co-writing sessions over lockdown—they finally paid off and I don't think I would've got this book done without them! Thank you, my favourite chaotic gals, for making me smile during the toughest times. Your belief in me fuelled my belief in myself.

I'd like to thank my interviewees for agreeing to speak to me and for sharing their personal stories, hot takes and useful insights: Beulah Davina, Charlotte Mensah, Dominique Lescott, Ebuni Ajiduah, Jamelia Donaldson, Lekia Lee, Michelle De Leon, Ruby & Kate Williams, Sarah Adesikun, Simone Williamson, Stella Lucien and Winnie Awa. To every Black woman who took the time to complete my online survey and contribute to my research—I appreciate you.

And finally, Daddy. Our time together was much too short, but I know that you are watching over me, protecting and guiding me through life. I hope that I've made you proud. One day we'll be together again.

ABOUT THE AUTHOR

Zainab Kwaw-Swanzy is an award-winning Product Manager and holds a Masters in Mathematics from the University of Bristol. She leads initiatives to champion diversity, inclusion and equality in the workplace.

Zainab was part of the founding team of award-winning magazine *gal-dem*, and is a public speaker regularly delivering talks and presentations about defying stereotypes and navigating spaces that lack diversity. In addition to her writing appearing in *gal-dem*, Zainab is a professional model and has modelled for Superdry, Pantene, Adidas and more.

Zainab's accolades include: Winner of the Black British Business Awards 'Rising Star in Financial Services' Award 2020; named in the 2020 and 2021 INvolve EMpower top 100 Ethnic Minority Future Leaders List; and featured in The Female Lead 2021 Book showcasing trailblazing women across the world.